Jeanne A. Petrek, M.D., was the second woman to complete the surgical training program at Harvard University Medical School's Peter Bent Brigham Hospital. Formerly on staff at Emory University School of Medicine, Dr. Petrek is now on the staff of Memorial Sloan-Kettering, where she specializes in breast cancer treatment and research.

A Woman's Guide to the Prevention, Detection, and Treatment of Cancer

A Woman's Guide

to the

Prevention, Detection, and Treatment of Cancer

Jeanne A. Petrek, M.D.

Macmillan Publishing Company
New York
Collier Macmillan Publishers
London

MACMILLAN PUBLISHING COMPANY
866 Third Avenue, New York, N.Y. 10022
Collier Macmillan Canada, Inc.

Library of Congress Cataloging in Publication Data

Petrek, Jeanne A.
  A woman's guide to the prevention, detection, and treatment of cancer.

  Includes index.
  1. Women—Diseases. 2. Cancer. 3. Women—Health
and hygiene. I. Title. [DNLM: 1. Neoplasms—popular
works. QZ 201 P494w]
RC281.W65P48 1985   616.99'4   85-7089
ISBN 0-02-595940-9

          Macmillan books are available at special discounts
            for bulk purchases for sales promotions, premiums,
          fund-raising, or educational use. For details, contact:

                    Special Sales Director
                    Macmillan Publishing Company
                    866 Third Avenue
                    New York, N.Y. 10022

          10 9 8 7 6 5 4 3 2 1

          Printed in the United States of America

To my parents, Emily and John Petrek

Contents

Acknowledgments

Many thanks to my research assistant, Phylis Austin, whose constant attentiveness and dedication to the realization of this work both smoothed and lightened the task, and to Michael Budowick of Emory University for the contribution of his illustrations.

I am especially grateful to my husband for painstaking and meticulous editorial assistance.

Introduction

The goal of this book is to inform women about important aspects of the most common cancers. The text has developed from questions and general discussions in the office of three groups of people: those with a particular cancer, those under evaluation, and the relatives and friends of cancer patients. The book contains discussions of some malignancies that I, as a cancer surgeon, have never treated; for these, I have relied upon colleagues and medical texts.

Each chapter focuses on a specific form of cancer, with references to:

- *The nature and normal functions of the affected bodily structures.* While this information may be generally known in many instances, in others, such as pancreas or larynx, some background is necessary.
- *Familial tendency.* Most patients whose relatives have had cancer overestimate their own risk. In fact, cancers differ greatly as to the susceptibility of relatives. For example, the daughter of a woman who has had cancer arising independently in both breasts at a premenopausal age is thought to have at least a 50 percent chance of developing breast cancer in her own lifetime, while there seems to be no increased risk if her mother has had pancreas cancer at any age.
- *Causes and associated factors.* In some instances, causation has been

established. For example, while an injury to the breast does not cause cancer, X rays of the breast may. The risks with X rays rise with increasing doses and the younger age of the patient. Japanese women exposed to radiation from the atomic bomb at middle age showed no detectable increase in breast cancer; on the other hand, teenagers living in the area and exposed to the same amount of radiation had a significant number of breast cancers. In other instances, certain factors are known to be associated with the cancer, but have not been established as causes. For example, while particular diets have characterized patients with higher or lower risks of colon cancer, it remains unclear how various substances in the diet may actually cause or inhibit the disease.

- *Prevention* Most women realize that not smoking will prevent the vast majority of lung cancers. However, a significant proportion of bladder, esophagus, and head and neck cancers can also be prevented by not smoking. The latest studies show that not smoking may lessen even the chances of cervix cancer. Other factors involved in the prevention of cancer are also discussed, including vitamin A (lung cancer), birth control pills (ovarian cancer), diaphragm usage (cervix cancer), dietary fiber (colorectal cancer), and vitamin C (stomach cancer).
- *Early and subsequent symptoms* Most people fail to realize that virtually no early cancer in any organ causes pain. Pain is common only in later stages. Cancers vary widely as to the number and kinds of other symptoms they may cause; by the same token, it is important to recognize that a symptom of cancer may be a symptom of another ailment altogether, and that only a doctor can make the proper diagnosis.
- *Detection and diagnostic tests* Whether it is human nature or fear of cancer, patients invariably imagine that tests and treatments will be worse than they actually are. Information enables one to face an event without the greatest fear—fear of the unknown.
- *Treatment* At one time, the discussion of treatment was limited to the one procedure that *had to be done.* Nowadays, patients question the need for, and choice of, treatment, and the possible risks and disabilities. Overtreatment is now considered almost as undesirable as undertreatment.

Physicians who inform their patients fully aren't merely being nice; they are obeying the law. The courts determined in 1972 *(Canterbury* v. *Spence)* that "doctors must disclose everything . . . they would expect the average reasonable person to consider material to a decision to undergo the proposed treatment. . . . An item of information is material if . . . it would cause a patient to refuse the recommended treatment." It is important to keep in mind that research on all forms of cancer is ongoing, and that a number of treatments are considered experimental primarily because the studies of their long-term effects have not been finished as yet.

As is apparent, I have not dealt with the psychological dimensions of cancer. They loom large in every doctor's practice and have been the subject of extensive discussion. For that reason, I refer the reader to the bibliography for supplemental reading.

It is my firm belief that information dispels the greatest fear—that of the unknown. Such fear can cause delay in seeking a physician for evaluation of suspicious symptoms. In 1938 a key study found that sheer ignorance of the meaning of a particular symptom was the most common cause for delay in diagnosis and treatment of cancer. Since then, fear and other psychological factors have played an increasingly important role. Recent reports have also cited unrealistic fears of mutilation, denial or repression of clear symptoms, and fatalism ("Once you have cancer, all hope is gone"). People fear cancer because they fear pain, disfigurement, disruption of normal activities and work, and ultimately, because they fear death. However, even when these fears are realistic, information is helpful; the facts about diagnosis and treatment are more encouraging than might be supposed, due largely to recent dramatic advances fueled by research.

In this century, the medical profession has come far in eradicating communicable diseases and dealing with trauma. Clearly, the next threshold to be reached is in the area of preventive medicine. In this area, patients must become equal partners with their physicians as they take action designed to prevent the occurrence of disease and disability. In *A Woman's Guide to the Prevention, Detection, and Treatment of Cancer*, my goal has been to provide women—traditionally the caretakers of family health and well-being—with the information they need to make intelligent health-care decisions for the long as well as the short term.

A Woman's Guide to the Prevention, Detection, and Treatment of Cancer

Breast Cancer

Perhaps because the breast is more external than other organs, its diseases—mainly malignancy and infection—have been described in ancient history books and portrayed in ancient art. The ancient Egyptians, for example, wrote about breast cancer, as evidenced in the Edwin Smith Medical Papyrus (about 2500 B.C.). There is also a piece of stone statuary, dating from roughly the time of Christ, that graphically depicts a breast in the late stages of cancer.

Cancer of the breast is exceptionally common and will affect almost 10 percent of all American women. One out of eight cancers in women develops in this organ. Yet it is not, so far as one can tell, as much an epidemic as many women's magazines would suggest. Even as recently as several decades ago, breast cancer, and the breast in general, were not discussed, probably because of lingering post-Victorian inhibitions. Accordingly, the greater attention now paid to breast cancer creates the impression of an increase in its occurrence. The incidence of breast cancer in the United States appears not to have changed appreciably since the 1930s, when good public health records were first kept, and numbers about 120,000 cases each year.

Although breast cancer in women under forty is much in the news, it is more a disease of the elderly. The occurrence of breast cancer increases steadily with age and is almost eight times more common in women aged seventy-five to eighty than in those aged thirty-five to forty.

SYMPTOMS OF BREAST CANCER

- Lump or nodule in the breast.
- Rarely, discharge from nipple.
- Skin changes, including dimpling.
- Shape changes.

SYMPTOMS

The most common and obvious symptom of breast cancer is a lump or thickening of breast tissue. However, what is commonly referred to as a "lump" can also be the result of fibrocystic disease. It is actually preferable to speak of "fibrocystic changes." Physical examinations for employment or insurance purposes reveal that more than 50 percent of presumably healthy women have irregular breasts with lumps. A situation involving so great a percentage can hardly qualify as a disease or abnormality. Curiously, it might be more correct to assume that the minority of women with smooth, soft breasts, free from any lumpiness, are those with the abnormality!

The category of fibrocystic changes (often called "benign breast disease") involves at least nine different kinds of cellular patterns, as seen microscopically. Autopsy studies have shown that, even among women who did not have lumps big enough to feel, 90 percent had fibrocystic changes that could be identified as such upon microscopic examination. For the layperson, however, the lumps large enough to be felt fall into two groups: the fibrous, or solid rubbery tissue, and the cystic, or fluid-filled lumps.

In most cases, fibrocystic changes involve some amount of lumpiness and some pain, both of which are worse immediately before the menstrual period. But the presence of the lumps and pain need not coincide. I have patients with severe soreness and pain, but without much lumpiness. This pain can persist through the whole menstrual cycle and be so severe that the woman cannot tolerate jarring her breasts, as she would when jogging or even walking quickly. Then again, I have patients whose breasts feel as if they contain different-sized marbles, but who have little or no pain. The discrepancy between the physical conditions and symptoms is puzzling, and no one understands it.

Like malignancies that occur in other organs, breast cancers begin from a single cell and can develop in either the fibrocystic (lumpy)

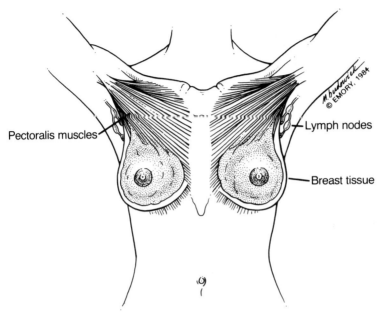

The breasts

or the smooth areas of the breast. Fibrocystic changes, however, are an obstacle to trustworthy breast examination, as benign lumps might make an adjacent cancer more difficult to feel. More important and worrisome than the mere presence of lumps or the pain is the concern many women have that these fibrocystic changes may turn into breast cancer. Be assured, however, that a benign lump cannot turn malignant.

Is there any association between fibrocystic changes and the later occurrence of breast cancer? Several research projects have kept track of women for many years after breast biopsy and diagnosis of fibrocystic lumps. The number of women in these studies who later developed breast cancer is about twice as high as the number never biopsied and diagnosed as having fibrocystic changes. However, twice the average risk is small, when compared, for example, to the risk of a woman who has a strong family background of breast cancer.

Unfortunately, drugs for fibrocystic changes are either ineffective or have major side effects. Therefore, drug treatment is recommended in only a small percentage of patients and then usually only in those whose pain is severe enough to interfere with normal activities. Since all researchers agree that fibrocystic changes are somehow related to hormones, the specific drugs used for the condition usually work by hormonal interaction. An example is vitamin E—which, in the high dosages needed for fibrocystic treatment, should be considered more a medicine than a vitamin. According to researchers, this vitamin may work by altering the adrenal hormones. Though vitamin E treatment brings improvement to less than half the women with fibrocystic changes, there are no side effects beyond an oily skin and scalp. Alpha-tocopheral (a form of vitamin E) is taken in doses of 600 I.U. (international units, a standard unit of measure) daily for eight weeks. This is a simple over-the-counter drug, with limited usefulness. But given its lack of side effects, it may be helpful in treating breast pain—as long as a physician finds only benign breast changes.

Beyond vitamin E, there are two drugs which, through action on hormones, more effectively decrease lumpiness, though at the cost of significant side effects. When these drugs' possible side effects—including slight masculine changes with Danocrine, and nausea, dizziness, and so on with bromocriptine mesylate—are explained, the patient tends to reevaluate how severe the pain really is. Both are prescription drugs, and Danocrine is quite expensive, in the range of $80 to $150 per month, depending on the dosage.

WHO IS AT RISK?

That breast cancer arises from breast tissue is not necessarily the truism it might seem. Breast tissue consists only of the milk-forming cells and the milk-carrying ducts, of which everyone has about the same amount. It would be as likely for the thyroid to differ in size from woman to woman as it would be for the amount of breast tissue. It is the breast's fat and connective tissue that varies and results in differing breast sizes. As the amount of true breast tissue is rather constant, susceptibility to cancer exists irrespective of breast size. Therefore, a woman with large breasts is no more likely to have breast cancer than a woman with small breasts.

In order to prevent a disease, one must have a good idea of its causes. Unfortunately, breast cancer has no known cause, as does, for instance, lung cancer (smoking). Of course, there are some associated factors, and people who possess these factors have a higher incidence of breast cancer; still, it is unclear to what extent such factors may operate either individually or collectively in causing the disease.

Does Breast Cancer Run in Families?

There may be a family or genetic association. I say "may" because families often have similar hormonal patterns or, for that matter, the same common diet. In such cases, the increased risk in certain families is not genetic as much as it is hormonal or caused by other common factors. At any rate, we know that the closer the relative, and the earlier the cancer in that relative's life, the greater the risk to their kin. In the case of identical twins, if breast cancer occurs in one, a substantial risk exists for the other.

Almost every woman will have some cousin or great-great-aunt who has had breast cancer; because this is such a common disease it is unusual to have none whatever in the family. The risk increases if the closest relatives (mother, sister, daughter) have had breast cancer, becoming almost three times the average risk. Risk also increases if the close relative's malignancy occurred before menopause. If the afflicted relative had cancer in both breasts, arising independently (that is, not starting in one breast and spreading to the other), the risk is even higher. The mother, sister, or daughter of a woman who has had premenopausal breast cancer developing in both breasts has about a 50 percent chance of developing breast cancer in her lifetime.

Hormones and Breast Cancer

It is clear that breast cancer has various hormonal associations: (1) a decreased risk of breast cancer occurs if the ovaries are removed at an early age; (2) an increased risk occurs if the menstrual periods begin earlier in life than for the average adolescent; (3) an increased risk occurs if there is a late menopause; and (4) a decreased risk occurs if the first full-term pregnancy is at an early age (in the early twenties or before).

The first three factors suggest a relationship between the greater number of menstrual cycles in a woman's life and an increased risk of breast cancer. As regards the fourth factor, there appears to be some phenomenon that depends upon the time in one's life when a full-term pregnancy—or a longer period when combined with breast feeding—interrupts the usual monthly cycles. A pregnancy ending in the first or early second trimester appears of inadequate duration to cause any change in risk factors, regardless of the woman's age at pregnancy.

That a full-term pregnancy early in life seems protective is perhaps due to the sensitive young age at which interruption of the menstrual cycles occurs. During pregnancy, the estrogen level does not fluctuate monthly and is higher than at any other time in a woman's life. Unfortunately, exactly how this hormonal state could decrease risk if it occurs early in life and increase risk if it occurs late is unknown.

Women who have never been pregnant are at greater risk than those who have been pregnant. And women in their late thirties who have a first full-term pregnancy increase their breast cancer risk, even over the never pregnant. In looking at the statistical extremes, a woman who has her first child after age thirty-five has at least three times the risk of a woman who has her first child before age eighteen.

The recent data about the long-term use of birth control pills and breast cancer may fit into the general theory. With birth control pills, even though one does have menstrual bleeding, the overall amount of the monthly hormonal fluctuations that would naturally occur is significantly reduced. Studies show that long-term pill users appear to have a slightly decreased incidence of breast cancer.

Caffeine, Breast Cancer, and Fibrocystic Changes

The relationship between high caffeine intake and breast cancer has been in the news since the late seventies, when researchers at Ohio State University first reported the association. The line of reasoning is: Caffeine increases a substance, cyclic AMP, that is almost universally present within cells and influences cellular metabolism. This increase of cyclic AMP is partly responsible for the certain "buzz" or energetic feeling one gets after consuming coffee or some other source of caffeine.

The Ohio State researchers measured the amount of cyclic AMP in normal breast tissue, fibrocystic breast tissue, and breast cancer. They found a higher level of cyclic AMP in fibrocystic tissue than in normal tissue, and a *much* higher level in breast cancer tissue than in fibrocystic tissue. This increase, however, may be the result rather than the cause of greater metabolic activity and cell division. It has not been determined if the process of cell division alone can increase cyclic AMP. In addition, this substance, so short-lived outside the body, is difficult to measure, and not surprisingly has been subject to debate about laboratory measurements. Besides caffeine, other factors that increase adrenaline, such as nicotine, various medicines, and distressing emotions, also increase cyclic AMP levels. Acting on the supposition that caffeine is known to increase cyclic AMP, the researchers asked normal women with fibrocystic lumpiness to abstain from all sources of caffeine. Later physical examinations found less lumpiness.

Since the time of the first study, another university conducted an excellent study that reproduced the Ohio State experimental methods as to the kinds of patients and lumpiness. This study could find *no* association between caffeine and lumpiness. Even more important, no researcher has ever found a relationship between increased caffeine and a higher incidence of breast cancer. In addition, two other studies found that women who had lumpy fibrocystic changes severe enough to undergo biopsy did not consume any more caffeine than those who did not.

According to my own experiments, caffeine in several different doses does not increase the rate of breast cancer in rats that are given cancer-producing drugs. Other laboratories have had similar findings. One never knows just how this information is best applied to humans, since animal breast cancer is not in all ways similar to human breast cancer.

Diet and Miscellaneous

Diet, in general, may contribute to an increased incidence of breast cancer, particularly one high in protein and animal fat and low in fiber, which is the typical American diet. This theory finds support in the high incidence of breast cancer in countries which share this kind of diet. Other countries, such as Japan, that have a high standard of living, similar to ours, but different diets, have a low incidence of breast cancer. In addition, recent data have shown that the typical American diet is associated with colon cancer, and it is known that women who have had colon cancer are more predisposed to breast cancer and vice versa. This may be so because a similar diet predisposes to both.

At one time there was a question as to whether hair dyes caused breast cancer, because there is a higher incidence in countries where such cosmetics are used, as opposed to countries in Africa and Asia where they are not. However, since breast cancer is not more frequent in beauticians, who are constantly exposed, than it is in other women in the United States, it is generally held that the high incidence is due to other factors.

There is no evidence that either mild, long-term trauma, such as nipple irritation which may result from jogging or bouncing sports, or sudden trauma, such as injury during sports (being hit in the breast with a tennis ball), has any influence on breast cancer.

Preventive Mastectomy and Reconstruction

Since there is no known way to prevent breast cancer, preventive mastectomy and immediate reconstruction is a much-discussed topic. Women who are at very high risk may choose to undergo removal of both breasts before the onset of cancer, usually with immediate plastic surgical reconstruction.

Such patients must be well chosen and well informed. Preventive mastectomy is offered mainly to women with the strongest of family tendencies—breast cancer occurring in both breasts premenopausally of mother, sister, or daughter. Preventive mastectomy is also important for those on whom a biopsy shows premalignant change—where the cells are abnormal but not yet malignant. Biopsies showing such atypical cells are less common than either those showing (benign) fibrocystic changes or those showing malignant cells. In addition, the procedure is sometimes offered to women who have had numerous biopsies, perhaps five or six, and whose breasts continue to form suspicious lumps, necessitating further biopsies. The indications for considering preventive mastectomy should be: (1) first degree relatives (mother, sister, daughter) with premenopausal breast cancer in both breasts; (2) previous biopsy showing premalignant changes; and (3) six or more biopsies and several years to go before reaching menopause (when the formation of benign lumps tends to decrease). I believe that reasons other than these should be considered long and seriously by the patient and her doctors. There are a number of women with the right background for this operation who choose to undergo it and later regret the decision. Breast surgeons often have altruistic and grateful patients who will show their reconstructed breasts to women who are considering such an operation.

The preventive procedure is sometimes a subcutaneous mastectomy, in which the skin, nipple, and all the muscles are left intact, and only the inner breast "mound" is removed. On the other hand, because the nipple is actually breast tissue—the exit point of the milk-carrying ducts—a better preventive operation removes the nipple as well.

Removing the breast with the nipple is called a simple, or total, mastectomy. Depending upon the size, shape, and skin condition of the woman's breasts, a subcutaneous or simple mastectomy is usually combined with the insertion of implants that refill the breast mound contour. The implants, which are made of silicone, are usually placed under the muscles of the chest (the pectoralis, etc.). This is a significant undertaking and involves many considerations, not the least of which are cosmetic appearance, complications of the operation, cost, and pain.

Despite such preventive measures, some risk of breast cancer remains because small amounts of breast duct cells are normally present in the tiny, delicate ligaments that reach into the skin itself. This means that only 90 percent or so of the breast can truly be removed, even in a thorough simple mastectomy, without injuring the overlying skin. It is theorized, then, that a woman's risk after a preventive mastectomy may be reduced 90 percent—or by the amount of breast tissue removed. After preventive mastectomy women will still require self-examination and physician follow-up.

Breast Self-Examination

Patients have many questions about the technique of breast self-examination, but it really involves little more than periodically feeling the breasts so as to learn which lumps are "normal" and have "always been there," and which may be new and potentially harmful. When a woman becomes serious about taking care of her body and decides to do a monthly breast self-exam, she should first undergo a self-training program. She should examine her breasts every day for several days in order to become familiar with the location of every thick or lumpy area. She should then be able to detect anything new. In fact, such women are often better at their own breast exam than a doctor, since a person feeling the same breast a thousand times can be better than a breast doctor who feels a thousand different breasts only once.

When a woman starts a breast self-exam she often wonders whether she will be able to tell if a particular lump is benign or not. I always point out that this is not for her to decide. When she starts the exams, a woman should see a breast doctor who will confirm that there are no suspicious areas in the breasts. This session will confirm the location(s) of existing thicknesses, and it is a good idea to get to know where one's normal lumps are, since they do not change much over the years. Afterward, her job is to report any new lumps to the doctor for diagnosis.

As you can imagine, the fibrous, or rubbery, scarlike tissue in the breast cannot possibly change quickly. Once one gets to know where the preexisting lumps are, no lump should suddenly appear, except for cysts, which are fluid-filled pockets capable of arising literally overnight. These cysts are usually slippery, round, and unattached, and it is very simple for the doctor to insert a tiny needle into the cyst, withdraw the fluid, and "collapse" the lump.

During breast self-exam, one should especially concentrate on the upper outer quadrant of the breast (i.e., the fourth part of the breast that is closest to the armpit). This area contains the greatest amount of breast tissue and accordingly develops breast cancer more frequently than the other three quadrants of the breast.

It is possible to practice breast exam on silicone-filled models. One commercial concern manufactures eight such models, and the woman is trained on the one that best matches her own breasts. Each breast model has several lumps—some fixed and some mobile—of varying sizes and depths in the tissue. Though this may be valuable for training, I still think a woman's own breasts are the best training device. Also, I doubt that silicone-filled models can adequately match different breasts. The fact remains that breast cancer most often arises and appears as a new lump, which is precisely what breast self-exam is meant to discover.

DIAGNOSIS

If a new lump is found, a woman should not wait before going to see her doctor. Although most—nine out of ten—lumps are benign, some are not, and the simple fact is the earlier one detects the cancer, the greater the chances for cure.

What does a doctor look for? A doctor suspects malignancy upon

BREAST SELF-EXAM SEQUENCE

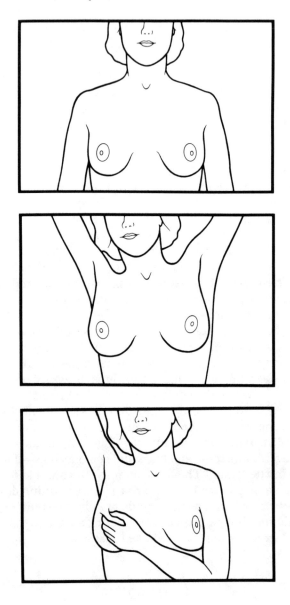

1. *Look at your breasts in the mirror for any irregularities*

2. *Look again with your arms raised*

3. *Feel your breasts for lumps, rolling the breast tissue between your fingers*

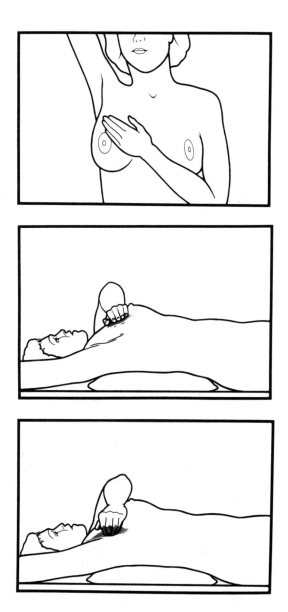

4. Press against the chest wall to find any lumps that may be fixed to it

5. Repeat the exam while lying down

6. Be sure to check in the armpit, as the tail of the breast extends upward into this area

physical exam if the lump is hard, feels attached to surrounding tissue, or is generally unlike other lumps in the breast. Benign lumps tend to be rubbery rather than hard. Cancer gets its name from the Greek word *cancer,* meaning "crab." The disease may have reminded the ancient Greeks of how a crab behaves when it tries to dig its legs into its surroundings and attach itself. This behavior is suggestive of cancer, with its "roots," or microscopic extensions. When a cancerous lump is manipulated, it is neither slippery nor movable, as is a benign lump, but feels attached to the nearby tissue. Doctors are also concerned with what is called a dominant thickness or lump. Although the lump may *feel* benign (is rubbery, seems unattached), if it differs from other lumps in the same, or in the other, breast, it should be biopsied. Occasionally, although a cancerous lump is not felt, its presence can be detected because it alters the smooth outline of the breast, usually by dimpling and indentation of the skin overlying the cancer.

Thermography

In addition to finding a lump by feeling for it, the only other reliable kind of detection is mammography. Before discussing the technique and usefulness of mammography, it may be best to say more about the advances in detection devices that do not employ X rays. First, there is thermography, which registers the breast's heat on a heat-sensitive device (some are similar to infrared film). As X rays are not involved, thermography may be considered as safe as being photographed. Thermography, however, is of little help in finding cancers, even though the underlying concept is good. Cancers usually give off more heat than the surrounding normal tissue because of their higher rate of growth and cell division; a cancer's greater blood supply also increases its temperature. Unfortunately, all this constitutes an insignificant temperature change, perhaps a fraction of a degree, and such small changes cannot be reliably registered. The amount of heat that actually reaches the skin level and can be imaged depends on the size of the cancer, its depth in the breast, and the size of the breast, among other factors. Thermography can find cancers that are reasonably large, close to the surface, and significantly heat-generating. But these are the cancers that could probably have been found months or years earlier by other means. In fact, one extensive study found a detection rate of 42 percent for thermography, compared to 92 percent for mammography.

There are several different tests using the heat sensitivity of thermography, including a home-device unit of heat-sensitive pads. The heat produces chemical and corresponding color changes on the pads worn inside the bra for fifteen minutes once a month. Color comparison from month to month indicates the heat changes from a specific area. This procedure is quite imprecise, and, in the absence of anything that can be felt in the breast, or seen on mammography, I wonder what conclusions to draw from more heat in one or another area of the breast. (Would anyone recommend removal of that part of the breast because it generated more heat than the month before?) Unnecessary anxiety could result in patients with an abnormal thermogram, when subsequent physical exam and mammogram are normal. Indeed, it was estimated from a nationwide study that for every woman with an abnormal thermogram and cancer, there are eighty or ninety women with an abnormal thermogram and no cancer.

There are many kinds of heat-sensitive devices widely available in doctors' offices. Although permitted by the Food and Drug Administration, evidence of their effectiveness in early detection is absent. One such thermographic device takes advantage of what doctors know about the abnormality of a cancer's blood vessels. The blood vessels of normal skin expand or contract depending upon the temperature. When one steps into the cold, for example, the skin's normal blood vessels contract to limit heat loss to the cold environment. When it is hot, however, or when one drinks alcohol, the skin's blood vessels expand to give off heat (causing the skin to look pinker). The blood vessels of a cancer do not have normal muscle coats and so they do not expand and contract. In order to capitalize on this natural process and highlight differences between malignant and normal tissue, one type of thermography requires that the patient sit naked to the waist in a cold room with both hands in ice water until normal skin blood vessels are maximally contracted. The difference between cancer and normal tissue is thereby emphasized even further, owing to the inability of the cancer's blood vessels to contract.

Still, thermography, or any kind of heat detection device, is ineffective in finding cancers that can readily be detected by physical exam and mammography. In addition, it is doubtful at this time that thermography can detect any important change in the breast, long- or short-term. For instance, suppose a woman has a baseline thermogram (i.e., when the breasts are entirely benign) and then submits to thermography every month for the next forty years. What are the chances that the woman will be alerted by any thermographic change at an earlier stage of breast cancer than by self-exam and mammography as recommended? Given the progress of current research, this may be possible within several decades, but for the present it must be ruled out. I am also concerned about the meaningless sense of security a doctor and patient may obtain from a "normal thermogram."

Diaphanography

Next, we have diaphanography (transillumination), a detection device that uses light. This technique was first used around 1910 and rapidly fell into disfavor, and for good reason: it was ineffective. Diaphanography involves examination of the breast illuminated by a bright light shining from behind it. This technique has been "jazzed up" in modern times by the use of powerful lights of different wave lengths.

The transillumination technique is effectively used in physical examination of the enlarged scrotum (the sack containing the testicles) to determine whether it is filled with fluid (hydrocele) or solid (hernia) contents. The transillumination is effective in scrotal exam because of the thinness of the skin involved and the limited and easily achieved objective of distinguishing a fluid from solid. For a breast exam, you might as readily examine yourself by holding a flashlight under your breast as rely on diaphanography.

Ultrasonography

Techniques using sound waves go by the name of ultrasonography and are useful for imaging many different organs. These tests present valuable information, with the further advantage of avoiding X rays or anything else that might be harmful. Breasts are examined using the same principles as in radar; inaudible sound waves, emitted from a source controlled by the doctor or technician, bounce back to a sensing device at different rates, depending on the density of the tissue. Ultrasonography, or "echo," is particularly effective in determining whether a mass is cystic (filled with fluid) or solid. If the mass is solid, however, ultrasound is not as accurate as mammography in distinguishing benign from malignant. The test requires the patient to bend over a container filled with warm water and immerse both breasts. There is no other contact, and certainly no pain or even detectable sensation when the sound waves pass through the breast.

Mammography

Finally, we come to mammography, which is recognized as superior to all current "-graphy" methods. It can find small cancers that are one-quarter of an inch, or sometimes less, and certainly does so before they can be felt by the most sensitive fingers of the most experienced doctor. Even so, mammography uses X rays and gives rise to the concern that the accumulation of many routine yearly checkups could themselves cause cancer.

As early as the fifties, mammography had acquired a bad name, primarily because of a study conducted by the Health Institute Plan of New York, which estimated that mammography could cause more

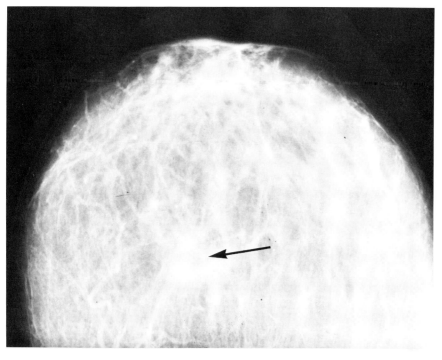

Mammogram shows small cancer undetectable on physical exam

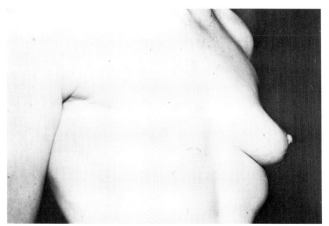

Standard mastectomy

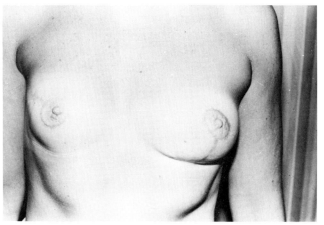

Post-mastectomy reconstruction. Right breast has been reconstructed; left breast has been lifted and rounded out to match the reconstructed breast

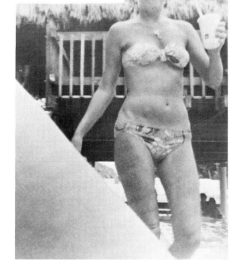

Patient following reconstructive breast surgery

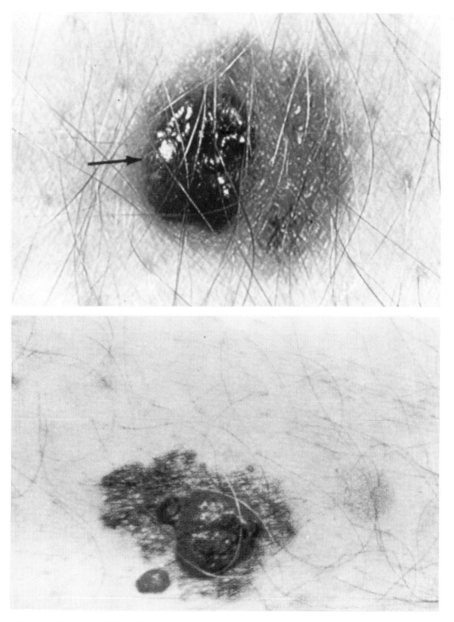

Early melanoma. Note the irregular borders and varying elevation of the moles. The extent of enlargement can be judged by the hair.

Various appearances of skin cancer. For the purpose of illustration, the cases shown here are more advanced than usual cases

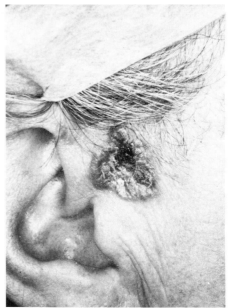

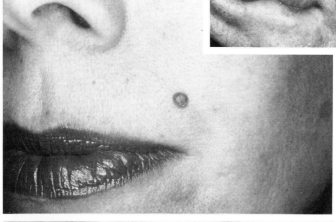

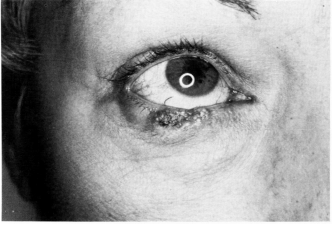

cancers than it found. But several important developments have occurred since then. First, the early mammography machines used much more radiation than they do now; second, mammography then was not as technically developed and simply did not find the smaller cancers it does today; and third, rather young women, even with low-risk factors, were exposed to mammography, in effect, for no reason. Nowadays, mammogram radiation is about one-quarter rad. (A chest X ray, for example, is under one rad; breast cancer treatment by X ray involves more than 4,500 rads.)

Probably because of the New York study, it was recommended that routine screening mammography, especially in premenopausal women, be infrequent. A more recent study, funded by the National Cancer Institute and the American Cancer Society, and based on 280,000 women in twenty-nine cities from 1973 to 1978, involved physical exams and mammograms for women who thought they had normal breasts. As opposed to the 1950s study, this one demonstrated that mammography was successful in finding early breast cancers in premenopausal women (under age fifty). Among the cancers found in these younger women, 90 percent were not detected by physical exam, but by mammogram alone. Premenopausal women have significant amounts of fibrocystic lumpiness that interferes, in varying degrees, with both mammography and physical exam. With technical improvements in mammography equipment, the interference has decreased.

American Cancer Society Recommendations for Screening Mammograms

Because of the proven effectiveness of detecting early breast cancer, especially in younger women, the guidelines for mammography have been changed. (See Table 1 for the 1983 guidelines revision.) A

Table 1. American Cancer Society Guidelines for Breast Cancer Detection, revised 1983

Age	Monthly BSE	Physician Exam	Mammogram
20–35	Yes	Every 3 years	0
30–35	Yes	Every 3 years	1 baseline
40–49	Yes	Every year	Every year or every other year
50 +	Yes	Every year	Every year

Note: The American College of Obstetricians and Gynecologists recommends that the frequency of mammography between the ages of thirty-five and fifty be determined based on risk factors, physical exam, and baseline mammography.

baseline mammogram is performed sometime between ages thirty-five and forty. The baseline exam confirms and documents the nature of the healthy breast at a given time for the purpose of comparison upon subsequent exams.

At ages forty through forty-nine, a routine screening mammogram is performed every year or every other year, depending on the physician's recommendation. Previously, no routine or screening mammograms were recommended for women in this age group. After fifty, the usual age of menopause, a mammogram is recommended every year. (Of course, if the patient or physician finds a lump or other abnormality on physical exam, a mammogram should also be performed.)

The area of least controversy is that of routine mammogram in the postmenopausal woman. Scientists know that X rays are less harmful to the breast after menopause than before, since X rays are most likely to cause a chromosome "mistake" (resulting in a malignant cell colony) in actively reproducing chromosomes. If tissue is dormant and inactive, as are the breasts with the lack of hormones after menopause, then X rays are not as capable of causing chromosome error.

In addition, with the hormonal decrease after menopause, fibrocystic changes and even normal breast tissue tend to shrink. This allows clearer mammograms and a greater probability of visualizing smaller cancers than in the premenopausal woman.

Conversely, the area of greatest debate has always been whether, and how often, routine screening mammograms (after the baseline) should be repeated in premenopausal women under age fifty. Most clinicians feel that if a woman is at high risk, a mammogram at least every three years is advisable for detecting any developments. Indeed, if risk factors are present (according to those outlined in the chapter), I agree that any woman is more likely to benefit from mammogram and early detection than she is to suffer the small possibility that repeated mammograms will cause cancer.

A mammogram is performed with detailed instructions from the X-ray technician. There are usually two views or films taken of each breast. For the horizontal view, the X-ray plate is placed beneath the breast. The woman is seated and the X-ray source is placed touching the top of the breast. The X-ray beam passes from top to bottom. For the vertical view, the X-ray plate is placed on one side of the breast and the X-ray source on the other; the view is from side to side. Both views involve some discomfort, as the plate must lightly compress or flatten the breasts for optimal imaging. There is no sensation aside from this slight and passing discomfort.

Though the mammogram is a great technical advance, one must

remember that it can detect only 80 to 90 percent of cancers of any size. Mammograms measure the difference in X-ray density between a lump and the adjacent tissue. If the difference is slight, the outline of the lump may blend with, and become indistinguishable from, the nearby tissue. Accordingly, lumps must be biopsied, even if the mammogram is normal.

Mammography has the advantage of visualizing the smallest of cancers, those that could never be felt. The procedure's disadvantages are X-ray exposure and a cost of $100 to $150 per exam.

Biopsies

Simply stated, lumps that could be malignant should be removed. To repeat, in general, a lump that arouses suspicion (1) is hard rather than rubbery, (2) feels attached rather than slippery, and (3) is unlike the other lumps or thicknesses in that woman's breasts. Since a lump does not necessarily have the same cells throughout, it should be removed in its entirety and every part of it examined under the microscope.

Any fluid-filled lump (i.e., a cyst) will be "removed" by the simple procedure of drainage with needle and syringe. It is useful to attempt such drainage with most lumps. The accurate diagnosis of fluid-filled versus solid is made quickly and inexpensively. If fluid can be drawn into the syringe and the lump disappears, the lump was a cyst. If no fluid is returned, the lump is solid.

How does the doctor remove a lump that has been detected by mammography but is too small to be felt by physical exam? Remember that such a lump, seen only on a mammogram, is embedded in fat and breast tissue, and, because of its small size—perhaps one-half inch or less—is almost impossible for the surgeon to see or feel during the operation. For this reason, the patient has another mammogram on her way to the operating room for the scheduled breast biopsy. At that time, the surgeon, or sometimes the radiologist, injects a colored X-ray dye into, or right beside, the lump. During the operation, the surgeon then merely removes the small part of the breast that has been stained by the dye. This localization technique is important for minimizing the amount of tissue removed.

After the stained tissue has been removed, a mammogram is taken of the specimen itself. This is to make sure that what had appeared suspicious on the mammogram also appears in the removed tissue. Since additional tissue will need to be removed should the suspicious area *not* appear on the specimen mammogram, the patient remains anesthetized. In most cases, however, one specimen suffices, due largely to the help afforded by the dye injection.

Local Versus General Anesthesia

As you can imagine, the time and manipulation spent in finding and removing the stained tissue (for lumps that cannot be felt) often necessitate general anesthesia. But for the actual dye injection in the radiology department, the patient is awake and a local anesthetic is used.

For lumps large enough to be felt, the best anesthesia, at least as far as safety is concerned, is local. This means that the skin where the incision is made and the area around the lump will be injected with an anesthetic, much like the one dentists use. The similarity to dental work is appropriate, since the pain with the injection, the painless sensation afterward of someone touching and working, and even the time required for the procedure are similar. (Many of my patients say that, however similar the two, they would prefer a breast biopsy to a dental procedure!) I give my patients 5 or 10 mg of Valium or a similar drug to be taken by mouth thirty to forty-five minutes before the procedure. When scheduling patients at 7:00 A.M. (requiring that they get up at 5:30 and take the Valium at 6:30) I often find they sleep through the procedure.

If general anesthesia is to be used, there are two possible approaches. One is the old-fashioned way, whereby patients arrive in the hospital the day before, have a chest X ray, electrocardiogram, blood and urine tests, and the biopsy the following day. Such extensive testing, however, is not always required for a brief procedure, and it is often unnecessary to tie up a hospital bed the night before a breast biopsy procedure in the case of a healthy person.

For minor procedures, such as breast biopsies, many hospitals have one-day service. The physical exam has been performed in the doctor's office previously. The patient appears at the hospital the day before the operation for blood, urine, and any other tests, then returns home, goes about her normal activities, and begins fasting from all liquid and food at midnight. After a good night's sleep in her own bed, she showers early and is admitted to a hospital bed. Following the biopsy, she is returned to her bed after a stay in the recovery room. When she is awake enough to walk, urinate, and drink fluids (usually four or five hours after the anesthetic), she can leave. She is not, however, completely back to normal, since slight aftereffects of general anesthesia will linger up to forty-eight hours. Accordingly, the patient should not be alone the first night and should not drive for at least forty-eight hours. Up to 18 percent of people report being uncoordinated (dropping coffee cups, for example) and perhaps 30 percent report muscle aches. Nausea and vomiting are also quite common the night after general anesthesia but, unless severe, are not a particularly good reason for an overnight stay in the hospital. In other words, one can probably be sick more comfortably within the privacy of one's own home, though the option always exists of spending the night in the hospital.

The advantage to the medical system is that of not tying up beds or nursing time. The convenience to the patient is that of spending most of one's time at home before and after a minor procedure. In fact, many medical insurance plans will pay 100 percent of outpatient surgery (which includes one-day service with general anesthesia) but only 85 percent of inpatient surgery (which includes overnight bed occupancy). The insurance plans are geared to encouraging cost-effectiveness.

Usually a woman can have the anesthesia she prefers. However, various factors about the particular lump or the patient's overall condition may dictate the choice. For example, a larger lump might be best removed under general. On the other hand, if the physician is quite sure by physical exam that the large lump is cancerous, it is possible to remove only a small part of it under local anesthesia to obtain a definite diagnosis of malignancy. (The rest of the lump can be removed in a mastectomy under general anesthesia at a later date.) In this situation, the patient continues to lie with an open incision under local anesthesia while a frozen section is performed to inform the surgeon whether or not enough tissue has been obtained to make an accurate diagnosis.

A surgical incision may be somewhat smaller if the patient is under general as opposed to local anesthesia, depending upon the depth of the lump. Vigorous manipulation for visualization in a small incision is of no consequence if the patient is under general anesthesia. Conversely, an operation under local anesthesia requires delicacy. (The difference in the scar length is so minor as rarely to influence the choice of anesthetic.)

The position of the breast allows for easy anesthetic and safe surgical access. The surgeon must have some experience in these procedures under local anesthesia, since slightly different techniques are required than under general. No matter how experienced the surgeon is with local techniques, however, at least twice the time—perhaps an hour—is required when the procedure is done with local anesthesia rather than with general.

Frozen Section Diagnosis

A frozen section is a quick means for evaluating the biopsy specimen microscopically within five or ten minutes of its removal. Because of the short time required for this test, decisions can be made while the biopsy incision is still open. Since additional tests may require fresh tissue, it is necessary to have the pathologist examine the removed tissue—both with and without a microscope—while the incision is still open and more tissue can be taken. The hormone analysis is especially important for determining cancer cell sensitivity to hormones (estrogen and progesterone)—information that can be valuable to later treatment.

I always have a frozen section performed on any tissue removed, regardless of the type of anesthesia and the low risk of any particular lump. If the lump is totally removed, the time of biopsy is the only opportunity for determining hormone receptors, which requires fresh tissue. The other advantage is that the woman immediately knows her diagnosis and need not wait a few days for the permanent section. The disadvantage is the cost, about $80, for the frozen section. This is in addition to the cost of the permanent section, which is always performed.

Scarring from Biopsy

The best scar, in terms of ultimate invisibility, is curved and located precisely at the junction of the darker skin of the nipple area and the lighter skin of the breast itself. However, it is possible to use this incision only when the lump is relatively close to the nipple area. Otherwise, an incision directly over the lump, wherever that may be, is used. Although there are several factors, including the lump's depth from the surface, that determine the length of a scar, one should expect the scar to be somewhat longer than the length of the lump itself. As is true with all incisions, a biopsy scar will not assume its permanent texture, color, and width for several months. This is particularly true for color, and it is not uncommon to wait six months or more for the reddish scar line to take on a normal skin color.

In addition, scars of the breast can widen, depending on their position. For example, the weight of a large breast, accentuated by the jarring motion of walking, tends to pull apart the edges of an incision. For any scar with this tendency, I recommend placing adhesive tape perpendicularly across the incision (sometimes called butterflies) after the stitches are removed. The weight of the breast and its jarring movement will pull on the tape and not on the scar edges. The patient can wash, swim, and play sports while replacing the tapes every week or so as the individual tapes fall off. It is difficult to know how long the taping should be continued. If a woman desires the smallest possible scar, she should probably continue for three or four months.

What to Expect After a Surgical Biopsy

There is usually little pain after the injected anesthesia wears off (after a few hours). What pain exists will be at its worst on the night of the biopsy. In fact, any kind of pain appears worse at night because of daytime preoccupations or distractions. Most patients take a mild narcotic, such as codeine, the first night, but then need only milder over-the-counter pain relievers. The breast usually hurts only when the incisional area moves, such as with walking, turning over in bed, and the like. I recommend that a firm support or athletic bra be worn day and night until the soreness ends, often within three to five days. Incidentally, with a biopsy under local anesthesia, the patient often drives herself to the hospital, has the procedure, and then drives off to the day's work, similar again to a dental procedure. (If she has taken anything like Valium, though, she should not drive.)

Care of the incision involves little more than keeping it dry for a certain length of time. The small amount of natural dried blood over the healing edge provides the best sterile dressing and should not be prematurely washed away. Though I recommend forty-eight hours, some doctors believe the incision should remain dry until the stitches are removed.

Biopsies Performed with Needles

There are two kinds of needle biopsies used for obtaining cells from a lump for microscopic evaluation: needle aspiration and core biopsy. Both can be done in the doctor's office. In the aspiration technique, a needle of the size used for drawing blood is inserted into the lump. A suction syringe then withdraws some cells that are prepared on a slide for microscopic examination, and the cells are studied for traces of malignancy. The main drawback is that the small amount of the sample may not contain the malignant cells, should they exist in a slightly different area of the lump. This is particularly true of smaller lumps, since the needle could conceivably miss the lump altogether and gather cells from the surrounding tissue.

If the diagnosis is "malignant," the technique has been very useful. If the diagnosis is "benign," one should pay no attention to it, since normal cells often remain as the malignant cells grow into the area. These benign cells may have been gathered from a malignant lump, assuming the lump was pierced in the first place. In other words, a benign result in this needle test should give no reassurance.

Many pathologists prefer not to use the aspiration technique in diagnosing malignancy. With this procedure each cell must be studied independently, since the few cells gathered by a small needle are not arranged in their normal pattern. A core needle (described below), or scalpel biopsy technique, obtains tissue with the cell pattern intact. This is helpful in diagnosis because there are important differences in the overall architecture of benign and malignant cells.

A core needle biopsy is performed under local anesthesia with a hollow cylinder needle about the size of a pencil lead. This small specimen, however, is still large enough for purposes of viewing some of the architecture as well as for studying the individual cells. Again, this technique can only be used on fairly large lumps and, again, it samples only a small amount of the total lump.

When Is a Biopsy Followed by Immediate Mastectomy Advisable?

Biopsy followed by immediate mastectomy is preferred by some women. If a lump has characteristics of malignancy, the surgeon can tell the patient that it is very likely malignant, though the doctor will always confirm the diagnosis by frozen section. If the patient is mentally prepared for a mastectomy after a biopsy with frozen section, she may desire to have it done this way. This is more often the case if she has friends who have had mastectomies, if she has obtained a confirming second opinion, if she has had the lump for a while and has been thinking about its treatment, and so on.

Most of the time, however, a patient is much better served—at least psychologically—by a biopsy followed by mastectomy or other treatment at a later date, when she has had time to reconcile herself to the diagnosis and to become familiar with various treatment possibilities. Though there is a medical benefit in biopsy with immediate mastectomy, in that one general anesthetic is less risky than two, if a woman is generally healthy and has no chronic illnesses, an additional anesthetic is of no consequence. Moreover, that most women are able to undergo a breast biopsy under local anesthesia removes this consideration.

The only other benefit of an immediate mastectomy is in eliminating delay between biopsy and treatment. It is theoretically possible that the incision into or around a cancer could send malignant cells into the opened blood vessels, thereby hastening spread to other organs. However, while possible in theory, data suggest that this does not occur. Studies indicate that the survival rate for women who undergo two-step procedures is no worse than for women who undergo biopsy followed by immediate mastectomy. Accordingly, there appears to be no harm in some delay between biopsy—whether the lump is partly or entirely removed—and mastectomy. (In addition, some women choose radiation therapy instead of mastectomy. In such situations, cancerous cells may remain alive for several weeks until destroyed by the radiation therapy.)

TREATMENT

Before treatment, the surgeon and radiotherapist will consider the possibility that the disease has already spread to other organs and will order appropriate tests. In other words, depending on the physical exam of the lump (including size, attachment to surrounding structures, etc.) and of the armpit lymph nodes, the examiner can predict the statistical likelihood of further tests' demonstrating spread. A simple blood test that analyzes the substances related to bone and liver function (two common sites of spread) is important to determine whether further tests, such as a bone or liver scan, are desirable. Unfortunately, the drawbacks of time, cost, and exposure to radioactivity are too significant for *everyone* with breast cancer to undergo the two scans. Therefore, the scans are recommended for those with a statistical likelihood of spread.

Bone scanning permits examination of the entire skeleton after an intravenous injection of a radioactive isotope. Normally, a uniform concentration should be seen throughout the bones of the body. An increased concentration is abnormal and may represent a tumor or old fracture. This test detects abnormalities sooner than an ordinary X ray. No fasting is required before bone scanning. With the patient lying in various positions, a scanning machine moves back and forth over the patient's body like a Geiger counter, and detects radiation emitted by the skeleton. The bone scan is performed two or three hours after injection of the radioactive material and takes thirty to forty-five minutes.

A liver scan is very similar, except that the scanning device passes over the right upper part of the abdomen while the patient assumes various positions. Neither scan should be performed during pregnancy, since the radioactive dose, though minimal, may be harmful to an unborn child.

The number of days spent in the hospital varies little with the two most common kinds of breast cancer treatment—modified radical mastectomy and lumpectomy with armpit lymph node removal and radiation therapy. Both require stays of five to eight days following surgery. With either treatment, less than 10 percent of patients will experience some degree of arm swelling. (The percentage is reported higher after a radical mastectomy.) The cause of arm swelling is not well understood and depends partly on obesity, the extent of the lymph node removal, whether X-ray treatment accompanies surgery, as well as other factors. However, swelling appears to depend even more on the postoperative care of the arm. With the lymph nodes removed, any infection in that limb cannot be cleared as quickly as normal. Moreover, recurrent infection tends to block the remaining lymph channels with the back-up fluid, resulting in visible swelling. By the term infection, I mean virtually any break in the skin barrier, such as occurs with an insect bite when scratched too hard, with cutting the cuticles during a manicure, with biting hangnails, with scratches from plants or bushes, etc. In fact, florists and gardeners seem to have the worst problem with postoperative swelling. I advise them never to be without gloves and sleeves while working with plants.

Radical Mastectomy

William Halstead, whose name is synonymous with the radical mastectomy, was a brilliant surgeon. His descriptions of some common operations besides that of mastectomy are still followed today. Before Dr. Halstead's technique became commonplace, a breast affected by cancer was amputated quickly and in its entirety, with severe bleeding. Postoperative infection and a difficult postoperative recovery usually followed. Often there was a cancer recurrence at the original location within months—that is, if the patient survived the operation at all. In 1894, an article by Halstead described his technique for mastectomy. It included removal of the pectoralis muscles, the breast itself, and the armpit lymph nodes and fat. Halstead also advocated that each tiny blood or lymphatic vessel should be severed and sutured individually. This painstaking process took six hours or more, but avoided the problems and consequent complications of earlier operations. Not only did the patients recover sooner, but the cancer usually did not recur at the operated site.

The pectoralis muscle connects the collarbone (clavicle), the breastbone (sternum), and nearby ribs with the upper arm bone (humerus). Even in a thin, unmuscular woman, the pectoralis muscle is thick. It covers the chest's upper ribs, fills out the contour under the collarbone, and creates the normal outline near the armpit where the arm joins the body.

Accordingly, removal of the pectoralis results in (1) decreased arm strength when bringing the arm across and in front of the body, (2) a depressed area, through which the upper ribs' outline shows on the chest, and (3) a deformed area where the arm joins the body. Besides the strength and body contour defects, the scars may be long and extend onto the shoulder.

Why was it necessary for Halstead to do such an extensive operation? The answer is partly to be found in his daily log. Halstead practiced over eighty years ago, in an era when women kept even their calves covered by long skirts. Breast disease was hidden. Ether, the first general anesthetic, had been discovered only forty years previously, and its use was not widespread. Operations were thought of as

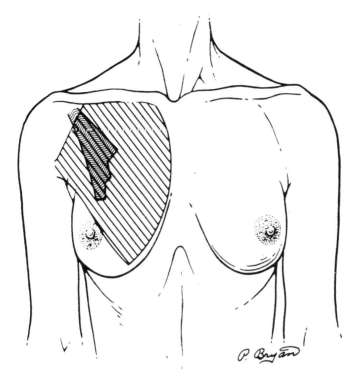

Chest wall muscles. Straight lines represent the pectoralis major muscle; wavy lines, the pectoralis minor muscle. Both muscles are removed in the radical mastectomy.

the last desperate attempt. For these reasons, among others, women arrived for treatment with massive cancers. According to his logbook, Halstead considered "small" the seven- to eight-inch tumors that he regularly saw.

Simply stated, Halstead created an extensive operation for an extensive disease. The pectoralis muscle was removed because it was often invaded and/or because its absence made removal of the large armpit lymph nodes easier. The long-term survivals of these advanced patients proved the effectiveness of his mastectomy. The results were better than any before his time and are, even by today's standards, quite respectable. In fact, a small number of patients today still arrive for treatment with advanced cancers attached to the pectoralis. For them, a Halstead (radical) mastectomy, with chemotherapy and/or radiation therapy, is usually best.

The number of radical mastectomies for American women has decreased dramatically over a short period of time. The records of the

American College of Surgeons show that the percentage of radical mastectomies was 45 percent in 1972, 22 percent in 1977, and 3 percent in 1981. The most recent survey included almost 20,000 women with breast cancer diagnosed in 1981. Women are now diagnosed with smaller cancers requiring less extensive surgery, and may themselves be partly responsible for this change away from radical mastectomies.

Modified Radical Mastectomy

In the late forties, as women began arriving at their doctors' offices with somewhat smaller breast cancers, surgeons devised the modified radical mastectomy. This procedure removes the breast, fat, and lymph nodes in the armpit, but preserves the pectoralis muscle. The inside tissue of the breast is removed, and the skin is kept largely intact to be sewn down upon the chest by way of reattaching the skin edge. With no muscles removed, the arm is as strong as before the procedure. The front contour under the collarbone and side contour at the armpit also remains normal. In addition, depending somewhat upon the cancer's site in the breast, the incision can be kept low, often at nipple level, and horizontal, so that it will not show when low cut dresses are worn. As removing the armpit fat and lymph nodes produces no visible change in the underarm area, the defect in a modified radical mastectomy is limited to the missing breast mound. The shoulder and upper chest appear perfectly normal halfway to the waist where the breast begins to slope.

The modified radical mastectomy is the most common operation today for breast cancer. According to three surveys conducted by the American College of Surgeons the number of modified radical mastectomies has increased: from 26 percent in 1972 to 58 percent in 1977 and 78 percent in 1981.

Extended Radical Mastectomy

This procedure, also called the Urban mastectomy after the surgeon who popularized it, was practiced during the fifties for breast cancers originating on the inner side of the breast nearer the breastbone (sternum) than the armpit. In addition to removing all the tissue included in the radical mastectomy, this procedure removed one-inch segments of the second, third, fourth, and fifth ribs near the breastbone. This was done to remove the small amounts of lymph nodes residing behind the rib sections. (The lymph nodes in the armpit were also removed.)

Almost all the lymph drains to the armpit lymph nodes, even if the lymph nodes near the breastbone are closer, as they are with cancers of the inner breast. If the lymph nodes near the breastbone are thought likely to contain cancer cells, X-ray treatment—instead of surgical removal in an extended radical mastectomy—is effective and usually performed. Three or four lymph nodes—but not the majority—may be biopsied, without removing the ribs or the muscle, at the end of a modified radical or radical mastectomy. Although a limited number of lymph nodes are obtained, such biopsy does not lessen the cosmetic result and may help the doctor decide whether X-ray treatment is indicated.

Simple or Total Mastectomy

It is, of course, possible to remove the breast alone and leave the lymph node area intact, a procedure known as a simple mastectomy. However, it is hard to imagine how this operation could be useful for breast cancer. Knowing whether the lymph nodes are involved is necessary for determining further treatment. Whether or not the lymph nodes are removed does not affect the appearance. Therefore, a simple mastectomy probably should be used only as a preventive or prophylactic procedure, as previously mentioned, for the woman at very high risk. Immediate reconstruction, with silicone implants placed under the chest muscle, is often performed. A nipple can be fashioned from the slightly darker and thicker skin of the upper inner thigh.

Subcutaneous Mastectomy

The other operation frequently recommended for prevention, the subcutaneous (literally "beneath the skin") mastectomy, involves removing only the breast tissue and leaving the nipple—even though the nipple is true breast tissue. The short incision is often placed on the under part of the breast where the lower bra line may conceal it. However, the top part of the breast toward the armpit is too distant from the incision for thorough breast tissue removal in that area. This, coupled with the fact that the upper outer quadrant of the breast is the site for half of all breast cancers, leads me to reject this procedure for preventive mastectomy. Needless to say, the subcutaneous mastectomy is even less appropriate for breast cancer treatment.

Most physicians, including myself, recommend simple mastectomy, rather than subcutaneous, for prevention because it allows more thorough removal of breast tissue. (A simple mastectomy is usually done through a larger incision because the nipple area is removed.) It might seem reasonable to let the nipple remain. However, because it has been detached from the underlying blood supply, it becomes lighter and sometimes discolored. This postoperative appearance is probably not good enough to justify leaving breast tissue. In addition, because the underlying nerve supply has been detached, the nipple has little or no subsequent sensation.

As noted earlier, breast cancer develops from the true breast cells.

Small amounts of breast cells are normally found in the delicate ligaments that reach into the skin itself. Therefore, even in a thorough mastectomy with thin skin flaps, a small percentage of breast tissue remains. In a subcutaneous mastectomy, depending on the thickness of the skin flaps, a much larger percentage, perhaps 15 percent or more, may remain. Does this mean that the woman's risk is lowered by 85 percent because that much breast tissue was removed? Everyone hopes so.

I have also seen various patients after a so-called preventive mastectomy who have 50 percent of their breast tissue remaining. Their surgeons probably felt that they would have a better cosmetic result with thicker skin flaps, which is true to some degree. To what extent are they now protected, if at all? For example, will the remaining breast cells concentrate the cancer-causing agents—whatever they may be—and will the remaining breast be as prone to cancer?

Partial Mastectomy, Quadrantectomy, Lumpectomy

As women in the 1970s and 1980s continue to follow instructions for early detection—self-exam every month and mammography as recommended—they are being diagnosed with ever smaller cancers. This suggests the desirability of a minimal approach involving removal of nothing more than the part of the breast with the cancer, surrounded by a margin of normal tissue. This partial mastectomy, though less extensive than other procedures, still requires the removal of the armpit lymph nodes, as well as X-ray therapy to the rest of the breast. The lymph nodes are usually removed through a separate, small (three inches or so) incision placed invisibly in the armpit. The lymph nodes must be removed in a partial mastectomy, if for no other reason than to determine that they were nonmalignant. If the lymph nodes prove cancerous, whether the mastectomy was modified, radical, or partial, further treatment in the form of chemotherapy may be recommended.

Following surgery, the remaining breast tissue, and sometimes the armpit, is irradiated over the next several weeks. The purpose here is to treat any roots (microscopic extensions) of the cancer, as well as any cancer cells that have moved through the ductal system or have arisen independently in another area of the breast. X-ray treatment to the remaining breast is considered essential. Studies find a 20 to 30 percent cancer recurrence in the breasts of women who did not receive postoperative X-ray treatment. The recommended treatment, then, is not limited solely to partial mastectomy, but includes the X-ray treatment of the remaining breast and removal of the lymph nodes. As you may imagine, it can sometimes be difficult to reshape the remaining breast tissue into a normal-looking contour after removing a relatively large cancer completely surrounded by a normal tissue margin. In the case of a small-breasted woman, the postoperative breast contour may end up cone-shaped and deformed. Partial mastectomies produce an excellent cosmetic result mainly when performed on patients with small cancers and medium or large breasts. (However, if the breasts are very large, it may be impossible to deliver the necessary radiation. Therefore, such a patient may also be advised to undergo a radical mastectomy.)

As of 1984, the best study available concerning full and partial mastectomies deals with women who had cancers approximately one inch or less in size. Half of the women have been followed for six years. The study shows no difference in the rate of survival of the women treated with partial mastectomy, accompanied by armpit lymph node removal and radiation therapy, and those who underwent a radical mastectomy. The women participating in the study were randomized as to either radical or partial mastectomy—that is, they had no choice of treatment. The study was performed on 800 women in Milan, Italy. (It is difficult to imagine such a large study being conducted in the United States, where most women know and ask for whichever procedure they want.) Randomization avoids such statistical problems as all young women (who, because of superior health in general, might be expected to do better) choosing the partial mastectomy treatment and all elderly women (who might have other medical problems) choosing the radical. In other words, the study appears to be a fair test of the two procedures among women with small cancers, and thus far the partial mastectomy group is doing as well as the full mastectomy group. However, six years may not, in fact, be long enough for reliable results, and some doctors maintain that cancer recurrence in the irradiated breast and its effect on survival remain matters for further study.

Surgical removal of the affected breast quadrant (or quarter-section) is referred to as "quadrantectomy." In a large-breasted woman, removal of a one-inch cancer with a safe margin need not include one-quarter of the breast; for women with small breasts, the opposite is, of course, the case. It is possible to skimp on the margin and depend more heavily upon radiation therapy to treat the microscopic cancerous extensions. This may be as safe as surgically obtaining the larger margin. To give especially high radiation doses to that area alone, the radiotherapist may insert tiny hollow tubes while the patient is under general anesthesia. The tubes are then loaded with powerful but short-distance radioactive isotope sources, calculated to give a rapid, high dose, but only over a short, perhaps half-inch, distance. After several hours to a few days, the extra radiation has been given only to the required area and the tubes are removed. Alternatively, depending mainly on the radiation therapist's preferences, about 25 percent more X rays can be given to just the small area of the former cancer.

In a lumpectomy, cosmetic results depend upon the amount of tissue removed, the dose of radiation, and the technique. Most women have what they would consider a good to excellent cosmetic result. The small percentage who do not, often have firmness and shrinking, or perhaps a deformity at the lumpectomy site. In addition, I occasionally see an unexpected psychological effect. Even though the patient was well-chosen and well-informed, and has an excellent cosmetic result, she becomes fixated about recurrence to the point of sleeplessness and depression. The affected breast, requiring frequent follow-up and attention, is a constant reminder of the possibility that cancer cells remain and may yet spread. Had she undergone total mastectomy, this concern would have largely been removed together with her breast. In the final analysis, however, it is distant spread rather than cancer recurrence in the breast that is incurable. Should the cancer recur in the breast (without distant spread), a total mastectomy would be in order.

Chemotherapy—as an Assurance

The treatments I have described are quite effective in preventing cancer recurrence in the breast and chest area. However, more than half of all women will have breast cancer cells recur in other organs, such as the bones or liver, in the several months to several decades after treatment.

Before detection and treatment of the cancerous lump, some malignant cells may have traveled through the lymph vessels into the armpit lymph nodes. In fact, lymph nodes contain cancer in about 40 percent of the mastectomies in the United States. Other malignant cells at the same time may have traveled through the bloodstream to reach other organs, such as the liver, lung, brain and bones. These cells are often too few to find by physical examination, isotope scans, X rays, computerized tomography (CT scan), or blood tests at the time of breast cancer diagnosis. Nonetheless, the cells may be present, and with continued growth will eventually make their presence known.

If the patient's lymph nodes do contain cancer cells, there is a substantial likelihood that other organs also contain undetected cancer cells. The expectation is that these cells will continue to reproduce and will eventually cause symptoms. Therefore, immediately after a mastectomy, when these cells, if present at all, are fewest in number, cancer-killing drugs injected into the bloodstream should be most effective. On the other hand, because no one can determine who has undetectable cancer cells and who does not, this program results in the unnecessary treatment of some patients with no such undetectable spread.

A woman will want to know all the statistics involving recurrence in patients with similar situations and make the decision about chemotherapy for herself. It is encouraging to know that the chemotherapy drugs for breast cancer are more effective than those for most other common adult cancers. When such additional, or adjuvant, therapy is used, smaller doses, and for only a several-month period, are given, in contrast to the situation where breast cancer has recurred and is under full treatment.

Even so, there are side effects, such as nausea, vomiting, and temporary loss of hair, that vary according to the drug and each individual's tolerance. This kind of chemotherapy program usually lasts several months. I find that many women lose only two days' work per month, especially if they have a desk job, as opposed to one requiring more activity. The drugs used for adjuvant treatment as well as for full treatment (for recurrence) are generally the same. They include cyclophosphamide (Cytoxan), methotrexate (Folex or Mexate), 5-FU (Fluorouracil), and doxorubicin hydrochloride (Adriamycin).

Hormone Therapy

The hormone analysis of the breast cancer done at the time of either biopsy or mastectomy will determine if the breast cancer is dependent on estrogen for a faster rate of growth. If the cancer is sensitive to hormones, then decreasing or otherwise altering the body's own natural hormones will, in most cases, result in slowing cancer growth. Women who have had a hormone-sensitive cancer growth should not take any hormones, such as postmenopausal estrogens, or even birth control pills. It is feared that the addition of hormones— even the small amount in oral contraceptives—could cause a hormone-sensitive cancer to grow. Many physicians, including myself, recommend against hormone or oral contraceptive usage after any breast cancer is diagnosed, just to be on the safe side. Most physicians also recommend not becoming pregnant after breast cancer because of the increase in hormones that occurs with pregnancy. The estrogen level becomes twenty to fifty times higher than during the nonpregnant state. There are, however, a few studies of small numbers of women who became pregnant after breast cancer and who did not seem to experience a worse course.

Interfering with natural estrogen effects is easier than one might think. It usually involves an antiestrogen drug (tamoxifen citrate) that has almost no side effects, although it does tend to be expensive. Before this drug was developed, the same effect was accomplished by surgically removing the ovaries and sometimes other hormone-producing glands, such as the adrenal and pituitary glands.

Reconstructions

After a modified radical mastectomy it is relatively easy to reconstruct the breast, as the missing breast mound can often be replaced with a silicone implant or bag. The silicone prosthesis is the same as that used for breast enlargement in a mammary augmentation procedure. After a modified radical mastectomy, the breast tissue and fat are absent, so that the silicone implant, lying immediately under the skin, often displays a visible circular outline. To avoid this problem, the silicone implants can be placed under the preserved pectoralis muscle, which hides the outlines and smooths the contour.

Unfortunately, the implant sometimes does not adequately match the other breast. The prostheses do not come in truly different shapes, but rather in various round sizes that match well only if the remaining breast is fairly round. Even so, plastic surgeons can often surgically "round out" the other breast, and regularly do so during the reconstruction operation. If significant plastic surgery is required to achieve the roundness, the patient frequently opts for preventive mastectomy on the remaining side, which means that both sides will be starting from the same point and the reconstructions will be easy to match. A preventive mastectomy is less extensive than a mastectomy for cancer, and it readily allows for simultaneous reconstruction at the same operation.

In a modified radical mastectomy, more or less skin is usually removed, depending upon various factors, such as the position of the cancer in the breast. Sometimes the remaining skin will be too tight for the placement beneath it of a breastlike silicone implant. To overcome this problem, a skin and muscle flap from another area may be brought to the mastectomy site. This is usually the latissimus muscle from the back, which provides sufficiently loose skin and a layer of muscle to hold an implant beneath it.

A particularly new and exciting, but complicated, reconstruction involves inserting muscle, fat, and skin from the lower abdomen at the site of the missing breast. In effect, the abdominal part of this reconstruction is the same as a "tummy tuck," in which plastic surgeons remove the loose skin and fat to tighten and flatten the belly. For purposes of breast reconstruction, the abdominal skin, fat, and muscle are reshaped and matched to the remaining breast in size and contour. Since the procedure uses natural tissue, the reconstruction is a softer structure than one made with the silicone implants. A woman need not be overweight to have the benefit of this procedure, because even thin women have the necessary surplus tissue.

Inasmuch as it is less than a decade old, the long-term results of the tummy-tuck procedure are unknown. Although the procedure is now being performed only in several university centers, it appears likely to become one of the more widely used reconstructions in the future.

Should every woman consider reconstruction as a matter of course? The advantages of a reconstruction are obvious when one considers the alternative—wearing an external bra prosthesis. The external breast prosthesis is a heavy silicone mold that matches the shape and weight of the other breast. The constant contact with the skin may produce sweating and sticking. If her breasts are moderate or large-sized, a woman usually finds she must either wear the prosthesis most of the day or else have a reconstruction to avoid the neck and back pain that may result from the posture and muscle imbalance caused by a heavy breast on one side alone. Therefore, the obvious advantages of reconstruction are not only cosmetic but physical.

Cancers of the
Reproductive System

The Vulva

The vulva is the term for the external female genital system adjacent to the vagina. Under a triangular cover of hair is the area known as the mons veneris, which covers the midline pubic bone. Between the legs, the hairy area divides in two and continues on both sides of the vagina for about three inches; these two folds are the labia majora (sing.: labium majus), which end close to the anus. The labia minora (sing.: labium minus) are the smaller folds of skin within the labia majora. They are hairless and much more sexually sensitive than the labia majora. The clitoris, the female organ that corresponds to the penis in the male, is located at the upper junction of the labia minora. The urethra, the point at which urine leaves the body, is the small dot or slit beneath the clitoris. These are the structures involved in vulva cancer.

Vulva cancers are "skin" cancers and as such may remind one of the harmless common skin cancers frequently found on the face and neck. However, while virtually no one (less than 1 percent) dies of these common skin cancers, the mortality rate of vulva cancer patients is 30 to 40 percent. There are, of course, differences between the two cancers. The skin of the vulva has a greater blood and lymph supply than the sites of common skin cancers. This may cause more rapid spread to lymph nodes or distant organs than is usually the case with skin cancers of other areas. In addition, a dangerous modesty seems

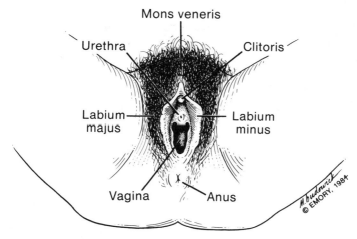

Mons veneris

Urethra   Clitoris

Labium majus   Labium minus

Vagina   Anus

External female genitalia

to prevail in older women—who are more likely to develop this cancer—resulting in a serious delay in seeking treatment.

The vulva, cervix, vagina, and anus are all composed of similar cells, and originate embryologically from similar tissue. Accordingly, it is not surprising that cancer in one of these areas predisposes to cancer in another. For example, as many as 10 to 15 percent of women with vulva cancer have had or will develop cancer of the cervix.

Fewer than 3,000 cases of vulva cancer are diagnosed each year in the United States, and the overall five-year survival or cure rate is about 65 percent. Most cases occur in the fifth and sixth decades of a woman's life. Yet a third of the patients are over seventy years of age, and, even of this elderly group, some 35 percent will survive five years or more with proper treatment. The ever-increasing number of elderly individuals will witness a proportionate increase in the occurrence of vulva cancers. While it is not clear just how many patients overall are "young," 15 percent of all vulva cancers treated at one cancer institute were in women under the age of forty. However, this number may not be representative of vulva cancer in general because cancer centers care only for patients referred to them, which can be a disproportionately high or low percentage of existing cases.

SYMPTOMS OF VULVA CANCER

- An open sore or lump in the vulva skin without symptoms.
- An open sore or lump with bleeding, oozing, itching, or pain.
- Occasionally painful urination if the open sore is near the urethra.

SYMPTOMS

About two-thirds of the vulva cancers are found on the labia majora. The earliest indication of vulva cancer may be an open sore or, less often, a lump covered with what appears to be intact skin. Occasionally, it may be itchy or painful when first noted. Some women notice the affected area only when there is bleeding, oozing, or painful urination. These symptoms, including itching and bleeding, are more likely to result from benign causes, hastened by postmenopausal thinning of the vulva skin, than from cancer.

Of all gynecologic cancers, cancer of the vulva is the most accessible to exam. While presumably the most amenable to cure for this reason, it is also one of the most neglected of cancers, with an average of ten to forty-one months of patient delay in seeking treatment. Bleeding has been reported in 31 percent and pain in 16 percent of patients for an average period of up to six months. Obviously, many months of treatment time are lost as the patient unsuccessfully tries ointments, salves, lotions, and other medications before biopsy and diagnosis of cancer.

Sometimes physicians add to the delay by prescribing various medications used for benign diseases, resulting in almost a third of the patients waiting an additional three months or more before correct treatment begins. Physicians may hesitate to biopsy the vulva when the patient is first seen because benign problems are so much more common. However, a greater degree of suspicion and wider use of simple biopsy are required for earlier diagnosis. After a short course of medication, biopsy should always be performed if the abnormality remains.

White Spots (Leukoplakia)

Leukoplakia (literally, "white patches") are white areas that may be thicker with folds and clefts or thinner than the surrounding normal pink skin. It is often not possible for a physician to distinguish visually between the various conditions and diseases—usually benign—that produce this white skin; final diagnosis must be made by biopsy and microscopic analysis. Leukoplakia appears not only in the vulva but also in the other parts of the body that have a moist membrane lining, such as the inside of the mouth and the anus. A few decades ago, leukoplakia was considered a definite precursor to vulva cancer. Since then, studies have been conducted that followed women with all varieties of leukoplakia over long periods of time, and they have shown that only a small number ever develop vulva cancer. Needless to say, any white skin areas must be biopsied, since some can be either malignant or premalignant. Only a pathological exam will determine the true nature of the leukoplakia.

WHO IS AT RISK?

Cancer of the vulva is primarily a disease of advanced age, often occurring in women of the lower socioeconomic groups and in association with multiple medical problems, such as diabetes, hypertension, and obesity. Whether these kinds of problems have anything to do with the cause of the disease is unknown.

Many chronic diseases and irritations of the vulva have been suggested as predisposing a woman to cancer of the vulva. However, chronic irritations seem to occur in everyone's life at one time or another. A history of syphilis or other venereal diseases, including genital warts and herpes, occurs in some vulva cancer patients, especially the younger ones, though there is little or no evidence that venereal disease predisposes to this cancer.

DIAGNOSIS

Diagnosis of vulva cancer is as simple as removal, under local anesthesia, of a sixteenth of an inch or so of skin, using either a standard scalpel or a circular knife. The amount of skin removed can be so small as to allow any bleeding to be quickly stopped, either by compression or by application of a chemical cautery; sutures are occasionally used. Only one or two instruments and ten or fifteen minutes are necessary for this office procedure. Because of the area's rich blood supply, an incision here heals in several days. Sexual intercourse might be resumed sooner than that. Because of the large variety of benign abnormalities that normally require biopsies for diagnosis, less than half of the biopsies performed demonstrate cancer.

TREATMENT

The natural progress of vulva cancer is generally that of a slowly growing lesion that spreads first to the inguinal, or groin, lymph nodes adjacent to the artery and vein of the leg and then continues to the pelvic lymph nodes adjacent to the major arteries and veins of the pelvis. The spread may be contained in these lymph node areas for long periods of time. If left untreated, an ulcerative process will destroy the vulva area, resulting in abnormal connections of the genitals to the bowels and urinary system. Hemorrhage and infection may also be expected late in the course. Distant metastasis (spread) to other organs is uncommon until very late in the disease, when distribution by the bloodstream may occur.

Surgery

Even though plans are individualized, the treatment of vulva cancer usually involves removal of all the fatty tissue and skin of the vulva, along with the lymph nodes of both groins.

Although extensive and about six hours long, the surgical treatment is not deep inside the body and is therefore not especially taxing for older women or those with health problems. As mentioned, the operation involves removal of the total vulva. The loose skin is merely closed upon itself. Afterward, the genital area is hairless.

Postoperatively, oozing and the collection of fluid at the site of surgery is minimized by suction tubes placed under the skin flaps for drainage. These are left in place for several days. Skin grafts are necessary only if so much skin has been removed that a simple incision closure cannot be made. Since operating in this area involves more bacteria than in other areas, infection is a common problem and antibiotics are usually administered. Swelling of the legs following lymph node removal, from the backing up of lymph fluid, occurs in less than 10 percent of patients; leg swelling is found more often in patients with more extensive disease who require both groin and pelvic lymph node removal. To prevent problems with swelling, patients are sometimes instructed to wear an individually made elastic support stocking during waking hours.

Because only the lowermost part of the vagina adjacent to the vulva is removed, the vagina itself remains close to normal size. And since sexual stimulation is more complex in women than in men, removal of a woman's vulva—which usually involves removal of the clitoris—does not necessarily mean that she will be unable to reach orgasm thereafter. Some women, particularly those who were formerly able to reach climax through vaginal stimulation, are able to reach orgasm even after vulva removal. Since the vagina is not greatly affected by vulva removal, a woman may conceive, and even deliver a child vaginally in some cases, after surgical treatment for vulva cancer.

The Lymph Nodes

As with other cancers, enlarged lymph nodes may indicate the presence of vulva cancer cells. However, a doctor may find it difficult to evaluate the size and consistency of the groin lymph nodes before the operation to remove the vulva, particularly in women who are very overweight. In fact, various reports indicate that 12 to 40 percent of nonsuspicious groin lymph nodes will contain cancerous cells upon study of the surgical specimen. In other words, cancerous groin lymph node spread will not be detected by physical exam in a certain number of patients.

Most physicians and surgeons believe that when vulva removal is performed without removal of the accompanying groin lymph nodes, the best therapy has not been provided. But since removing groin lymph nodes is a more complicated operation, removing only the vulva—if the groin lymph nodes are not enlarged—may be best for the small percentage of patients with multiple medical problems who are at high risk from a longer procedure. In addition, when the cancer is superficial, penetrating no more than a sixteenth of an inch, there is a negligible chance of spread and lymph nodes usually need not be removed.

Lymph node spread, whether to the groin or pelvis, occurs in about half of all women with vulva cancer. Lymph node spread is found in 10 percent of the cases where the cancer is a half inch across or less. If the vulva cancer is larger than three inches, lymph node spread is found in 60 percent of the women.

Some patients have asked why it is not possible to remove the groin lymph nodes only on the same side as the vulva cancer. This is an attractive idea since most cancers of other organs drain to the closest lymph nodes. The lymph vessels of the vulva, however, are numerous and arise from a fine, diffuse network covering the entire area. Numerous studies have revealed that lymph vessels from both sides of the vulva join together, and a significant number of vulva cancers drain to both sides.

As stated, groin lymph nodes are routinely removed in treating vulva cancer. About 8 to 15 percent of patients with cancerous groin lymph nodes experience spread to the pelvic lymph nodes also. This small percentage of patients must undergo surgical removal, through an abdominal incision, or X-ray therapy to treat the additional amount of disease. This extra procedure is more likely to cause permanent leg swelling, the more so in heavier women.

In Situ *Cancer*

In any form of cancer, the abnormal cells called *in situ* represent mild disease. *In situ* ("on the place") refers to cells that appear, under a microscope, identical to any cancer cell, but have not yet invaded the skin barrier, as an actual cancer does. In other words, *in situ* cells are as close to being routine cancer as possible, without actually attaining that status.

If only a distinct, or several distinct, separate spots of *in situ* cancer cells are present, it may be possible to remove only the spot or spots, plus a margin of normal tissue. Women who undergo *in situ* removal then need careful, routine follow-up for the rest of their lives because of the strong tendency for other *in situ* cells or actual cancers to emerge, mainly on the vulva, but also on related tissue, such as the vagina, cervix, and anus.

If the *in situ* change is extensive, and involves more area, it is possible to carry out a superficial removal of the vulva skin without also removing the clitoris or underlying fat, followed by replacement with a skin graft. Following this procedure a woman usually enjoys good sensation and normal intercourse with orgasm. In fact, sexual intercourse may be significantly improved in patients who have suffered from chronic vulva irritation with itching, oozing, or bleeding prior to surgery. With surgical removal of the affected skin, the irritation permanently subsides.

Radiation

Overall, about 40 percent of patients with spread to groin nodes can be cured. In the presence of very large, matted-together lymph nodes or ulcerated groin skin, a woman often undergoes radiation therapy prior to surgery to shrink the groin spread. If the surgery is done before the X-ray therapy, the healing surgical incisions may break down. Sometimes the best plan involves removing the vulva, irradiating the groin, and then surgically removing the groin lymph nodes. Because of the X rays' adverse effect on blood supply and healing, it is often necessary to bring tissue that has not been irradiated from a nearby area to cover the irradiated site.

X-ray treatment of the vulva itself has also been performed, especially in those women for whom surgery is deemed inappropriate because of general ill-health or specific disease. There are, however, complications, including infection, scarring, and breakdown of the skin, along with pain, causing frequent interruptions of the X-ray therapy.

Chemotherapy

So few patients have distant organ spread—the usual reason for chemotherapy—that optimal drug treatment plans are largely unexplored. However, cancer shrinkage has been noted with methotrexate (Mexate or Folex), cyclophosphamide (Cytoxan), doxorubicin hydrochloride (Adriamycin), and bleomycin sulfate (Blenoxane).

Nonsurgical therapy with topical creams containing chemotherapy agents in premalignant *in situ* areas was reported initially with great hopes. But subsequent reports have dampened enthusiasm because of significant rates of nonresponse and recurrence when response had occurred. In addition, the conscientious continued use of chemotherapy cream involves considerable pain.

Results of Treatment

With a tumor that is confined to the skin of the vulva, even if it has spread to the nodes (assuming the spread is minimal), the chance for survival may still be 60 to 70 percent. The size of the cancer, the depth of its surface penetration, the differentiation of the cancer cells, and the extent of lymph node involvement all enter into the predicted survival rates as well as into planning the appropriate treatment. If cancer returns in the vulva area, it can be removed again in almost half the cases. If cancer recurs in the groin area, it is much harder, and sometimes impossible, to remove. While 80 percent of all patients without lymph node spread survive more than five years, only 40 percent of patients with lymph node spread do so.

The Vagina

The vagina is the tube-shaped organ connecting a woman's external genitals with the cervix, which is the part of the uterus that projects an inch or so into the top of the vagina. The walls of the vagina are adjacent to the rectum in the rear and to the bladder's base and outlet (urethra) in front.

The vaginal lining is composed mainly of squamous (scaly) tissue similar to that inside the mouth. Also interspersed in the lining are glands that produce secretions. As in other organs, almost all vaginal cancers arise from the lining. About 80 percent of all vaginal cancers arise from squamous tissue, and more than half the women affected by squamous tissue vaginal cancer are over sixty-five years of age. Cancers arising in young women, the so-called DES (diethylstilbestrol) daughters, arise in the glandular tissue. The average age of these women at the time of diagnosis is nineteen. This cancer of glandular origin—called clear cell cancer—is rare, with only 275 total cases reported in the United States as of 1980.

There are fewer than 1,000 cases of vaginal cancer—of either kind—diagnosed each year in the United States, with about 400 deaths; the cure rate is roughly 60 percent. If one considers all female reproductive cancers (ovary, fallopian tubes, endometrium, cervix, vagina, vulva), vaginal cancer constitutes only 1 to 2 percent. Actually, vaginal cancers that have arisen from other organs and merely spread to the vagina are more common than cancers arising in the vagina itself. More than half the time, cancer arising from the vagina is located in

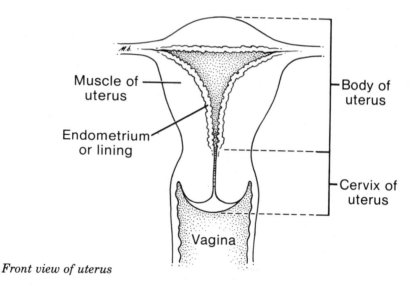

Muscle of uterus

Endometrium or lining

Body of uterus

Cervix of uterus

Vagina

Front view of uterus

the back of the uppermost vagina. The second most common location is near the outlet of the vagina.

SYMPTOMS OF VAGINAL CANCER

- Blood-tinged vaginal discharge.
- Vaginal bleeding.
- Burning irritation, frequency, and urgency of urination (with cancer in the lowermost vagina).

SYMPTOMS

The signs and symptoms of vaginal cancer are highly similar to those of cervical cancer. Vaginal discharge, often tinged with blood, is the most frequent symptom. Irregular spotting and postmenopausal bleeding are other common signs. Symptoms associated with the urinary tract—burning urination, frequency, and urgency—are more common than with cervical cancer. This occurs because cancers of the lowermost vagina are close to the bladder base and its outlet.

Unfortunately, the elasticity of the vagina allows cancers to become rather large before they are detected. Symptoms may be limited to discharge or bleeding, if anything. A large vaginal cancer is more likely in sexually inactive elderly women, who tend to undergo routine pelvic exams less frequently.

WHO IS AT RISK?

Vaginal cancer is so uncommon that few statistical studies have been made. At the same time, a woman who has or has had a cancer of the external genitals (vulva) or cervix, is predisposed to vaginal cancer because the tissue common to these three organs is similar and has a similar embryologic origin. As far as can be determined, vaginal cancer does not run in families.

DES and Its Uses

DES, which may be responsible for clear cell vaginal cancers, was developed in 1938 and became the first inexpensive, effective oral estrogen. It was used for many reasons, among them stopping milk production after childbirth, replacing estrogen during menopause, and controlling malignancies in the hormone-sensitive varieties of breast and prostate cancer. In the 1940s, doctors began to prescribe it to prevent miscarriages. Its use was frequent in the 1950s and early 1960s, mainly for pregnant women who experienced bleeding or other symptoms that threatened a miscarriage and for women who were known to have miscarried previously.

In 1971, however, the U.S. Food and Drug Administration banned the use of DES and other related drugs during pregnancy. Research published in that year established that women exposed to DES *in utero* had a greater chance of developing the rare vaginal cancer known as clear cell cancer. This appears to be the case with the mothers who took DES before the eighteenth week of pregnancy, when the developing genital tract in the unborn child is sensitive to drug-induced birth defects.

One to 2 million women already know they were exposed to DES before they were born. Between 1 out of every 1,000 to 1 out of every 10,000 DES daughters will develop this unusual cancer. Occasionally, the cancer does not occur in the vagina; rather, the DES daughter develops clear cell cancer of the cervix. In addition, DES can cause multiple benign abnormalities of the genital tract, particularly of the vagina and cervix. The infertility rate among DES daughters is significant, probably due to these abnormalities.

Do You Know Whether Your Mother Took DES?

As of 1984, women between the ages of thirteen and forty-four may have been exposed to DES before birth.

Use of DES was most frequent in the early 1950s. It began to decrease in the late fifties after randomized clinical trials showed that DES was not effective in preventing miscarriages. Finally, in 1971, the Food and Drug Administration banned the use of DES during

DES-TYPE DRUGS THAT MAY HAVE BEEN PRESCRIBED TO PREGNANT WOMEN

Nonsteroidal Estrogens

Benzestrol
Chlorotrianisene
Comestrol
Cyren A.
Cyren B.
Delvinal
DES
Des Plex
Dibestil
Diestryl
Dienestrol
Dienoestrol
Diethylstilbestrol
   dipalmitate
Diethylstilbestrol
   diphosphate
Diethylstilbestrol
   dipropionate
Diethylstilbenediol
Digestil
Domestrol
Estilben
Estrobene
Estrobene DP.
Estrosyn
Fonatol
Gynben
Gyneben
Hexestrol
Hexoestrol
Hi-Bestrol
Menocrin
Meprane
Mestilbol
Methallenestril
Microest

Mikarol
Mikarol forti
Milestrol
Monomestrol
Neo-Oestranol I
Neo-Oestranol II
Nulabort
Oestrogenine
Oestromenin
Oestromon
Orestol
Pabestrol D.
Palestrol
Restrol
Stil-Rol
Stilbal
Stilbestrol
Stilbestronate
Stilbetin
Stilbinol
Stilboestroform
Stilboestrol
Stilboestrol DP.
Stilestrate
Stilpalmitate
Stilphostrol
Stilronate
Stilrone
Stils
Synestrin
Synestrol
Synthoestrin
Tace
Vallestril
Willestrol

Nonsteroidal Estrogen–Androgen Combinations

Amperone
Di-Erone

Estan
Metystil

Teserene　　　　　　　　Tylosterone
Tylandril

Nonsteroidal Estrogen–Progesterone Combination
Progravidium

Vaginal Cream Suppositories with Nonsteroidal Estrogens
AVC cream with Dienestrol
Dienestrol cream

Courtesy of U.S. Department of Health and Human Services, Public Health Service, National Institutes of Health

pregnancy. Accordingly, women born between 1951 and 1953 have the highest incidence of clear cell cancer of the vagina. The incidence or frequency of this cancer appeared to peak in the mid-1970s and is now declining. Countries in Western Europe, as well as Canada, Mexico, and Australia have also reported clear cell cancer of the vagina among DES daughters. There were no cases reported in Scandinavia, where DES was not used in high-risk pregnancies.

DES Facts

The vast majority of clear cell vaginal cancers occur in patients aged fourteen to twenty-three years, with a peak at seventeen to nineteen years. This relatively narrow range suggests that, in addition to DES exposure, a factor associated with the onset of puberty is necessary for this particular cancer to develop. It is too soon to know whether some cancers will continue to occur in coming years as the DES daughters become older.

Among patients with clear cell cancer whose mothers' drug usage could be ascertained, about 65 percent remembered taking DES or related drugs, about 10 percent had taken an unidentified medicine to prevent miscarriage, and about 25 percent were certain that they had taken no medicine to maintain their pregnancy. Those women who thought that they had not taken DES or related drugs may have had faulty memories. Some of the mothers of daughters with clear cell vaginal cancer had no history of miscarriage nor any difficulties with pregnancy, and it is possible that DES may have been administered in the absence of a threatened miscarriage (e.g., to women with no particular health problems statistically predisposing to a higher miscarriage rate), without the mother's remembering or even knowing.

Investigators also wonder whether the presence of DES in food could by itself cause clear cell cancer in some sensitive individuals.

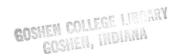

Since 1954, more than 75 percent of the cattle raised in the United States and some percentage of poultry had stilbestrol, used to fatten the animals quickly, included in their diet.

It should be mentioned that clear cell cancers of the vagina and cervix are believed to arise from the same kind of glandular tissue that would also give rise to endometrial cancer and to certain cancers of the ovary. Since DES daughters could develop cancers other than vaginal cancer, long-term follow-up will be necessary to detect an early occurrence of whatever cancer.

As for the mothers who took DES during pregnancy, there is little or no increase in general cancer incidence. There was only a small increase in the number that developed breast cancer, with 4.6 percent of DES mothers developing this malignancy versus 3.1 percent of similar women who never took DES. The increase in other reproductive organ cancers was equally small.

DETECTION AND DIAGNOSIS

To detect vaginal cancer, a pelvic exam, including careful inspection of vaginal walls with a speculum instrument, is most important. Although visible growths are the most common manifestation of vaginal cancer, early cancer occasionally appears as a small lump that can be felt even before it is seen. As unusual benign changes occur with great frequency in DES daughters, it is in the best interest of these women to be checked at centers specializing in such problems.

TREATMENT

In the earliest stage of vaginal cancer, a removal and reconstruction operation is often performed, especially for the younger patients. Other patients with early disease undergo X-ray treatment, both by temporarily placed internal sources and by external beam. For them, such treatment is as effective as surgery. Both procedures have advantages, depending on the location of the vaginal cancer. Because of their complexity both radiation and surgery should be performed at cancer centers, if possible, or at large medical centers with a special interest in cancer.

Surgery

Surgery for upper vaginal cancer consists of removal of the whole uterus (body and cervix), pelvic lymph nodes, and usually all of the vagina. If the cancer is uppermost in the vagina, it may be possible to leave half of the vagina, which will then permit sexual intercourse. Regardless of where the vaginal cancer occurs, the ovaries may safely be left in place when the uterus is removed. This is useful especially for young women, who have many years left before menopause. If external beam X-ray treatment to the pelvis is anticipated, the ovaries may be surgically moved from their normal position low in the pelvis to a location higher in the abdomen. In that way, when the patient undergoes the X-ray treatment, the abdomen and ovaries can be protected by a lead shield. Otherwise, the treatment would damage the ovaries and cause immediate menopause.

A vagina is usually reconstructed with skin grafts or with a combination of muscle, fat, and skin taken from the inner thigh. Sometimes a soft plastic cylinder—a dilator—is used to hold the vaginal sides apart while healing takes place. If the woman is not having regular sexual intercourse, she may need to use the cylinder once or twice a month, to avoid collapse of the vagina. Occasionally, an isolated loop of bowel is placed in the position of the removed vagina. If the vagina is shortened, with part remaining in place, as is likely with cancer of the uppermost vagina, then intercourse may require "positioning" (i.e., keeping the legs together during sexual intercourse so that the inner thighs create the impression of increased vaginal length). Since the vagina's removal also involves removal of the glands that produce lubrication, a lubricant may be required for comfortable intercourse.

Radiation

X ray can be used effectively in the early stage of vaginal cancer and is the treatment of choice for all later stages. Depending upon the exact location and the extent of disease at the time of diagnosis, three different techniques are used.

Intravaginal radiation involves insertion, usually under general anesthesia, of a cylinder applicator that spreads the vagina. The cylinder comes in different sizes, but is usually about 1½ inches in diameter, and has holes to hold the radioactive sources in place. The cancer-destructive rays of the radioactive isotopes, though traveling only short distances, have considerable power. It is necessary to keep the radioactive cylinder in place for twenty to forty hours. With this technique, as with the one that follows, enemas are given before placement. In addition, a catheter is used to drain the bladder, allowing the patient to maintain strict bedrest during the treatment.

Interstitial implant is a technique used for a variety of cancers, not just for those of the vagina. Under general anesthesia, narrow hollow catheters, the size of ballpoint pen refills, are placed through the cancer. The radioactive isotopes, manufactured onto a thin wire, are inserted into the catheters for short-distance but powerful treatment of the area. Then, after a certain number of hours, both the isotope wires and the catheters are removed, usually without requiring anesthesia.

External beam X-ray treatment involves treatment of the entire vagina and pelvic lymph nodes. Because the ovaries, bladder, and rectum are in the path of the X-ray beam, a side effect is ovarian failure and immediate menopause. It is still unknown if there is a risk to hormone replacement after such a menopause.

Aftereffects of pelvic irradiation, depending on the amount needed, include some degree of stiffness, narrowness, and dryness in the vagina due to scarring. Radiation, in general, may produce fatigue and nausea, especially if some of the intestines are irradiated. Because radiation destroys the vaginal mucus-producing glands, dryness is profound. A water-soluble lubricant, such as the one doctors use for pelvic exams, is necessary for comfortable intercourse. It is a nonprescription item, available over-the-counter at all drugstores. Major X-ray complications occur in less than 5 percent of patients.

Between 5 and 10 percent of all patients have spread of cancer not only to the pelvic lymph nodes but also to the groin lymph nodes. These are usually patients who have cancer in the lowermost vagina near the outlet. The cancer tends to spread, as a vulva cancer would, to the groin lymph nodes. It is often necessary to also treat the groins with radiation or surgery as a matter of course.

Clear Cell Cancer

Early stages of clear cell cancer can be treated either with surgery or radiation therapy. All other stages must be treated with radiation therapy. Surgery has the advantage of preserving better vaginal and ovarian function. However, some specialists disagree and believe that modern intravaginal X-ray treatment with internal radioactive sources is comparable, if not better. Vaginal clear cell cancer requires removal of all the vagina and cervix, or treatment of these areas with X rays, since any part of the area may be prone to recurrence in the future.

Chemotherapy

Because of vaginal cancer's rarity, there is little experience with the usefulness of various drugs.

SEXUAL FUNCTION AFTER TREATMENT FOR VAGINAL CANCER

Can a woman have a sexual climax after removal of the vagina? Usually the answer is yes. This is because the clitoris, as well as most of the muscles responsible for the contractions during orgasm, remains intact. The nerve supply to the sexual apparatus coursing through the pelvis is also largely intact, depending on the extent of the operation to remove the pelvic lymph nodes. Both surgery and X-ray therapy produce scarring of the vagina. Scarring, with consequent stiffness, dryness, and narrowing, is usually worse with X-ray therapy.

The Cervix

The cervix is the part of the uterus—similar in size and shape to the smaller end of a pear—that projects into the top of the vagina. It measures only about one to one-and-a-half inches at most. The cervix is separated from the bladder by a small amount of fatty tissue and the vaginal wall. The center of the cervix has a canal that connects with the interior of the body of the uterus, allowing the sperm to enter the uterus. If conception occurs, the central canal will be the birth passageway; if not, menstrual blood will continue to pass through.

In the United States, about 17,000 new cases of cervical cancer are diagnosed and 6,000 deaths result each year. One out of every fifty-eight women develops cervical cancer, which means that each woman has a lifetime chance of 1.7 percent. Although cervical cancer is the most common gynecologic cancer, it is surpassed by ovarian cancer as the leading cause of death. In a study of more than 10,000 patients, the median, or typical, age for diagnosis of cervix cancer was fifty-one years, meaning that half were in their forties or younger and half were in their fifties or older.

Cervical cancer almost always arises at the junction of the central canal and the outer side of the cervix. At this junction, the glandular tissue of the canal becomes squamous; that is, the tissue changes from that characterizing the inside of the uterus (glandular) to that characterizing the outer cervix and vagina (squamous). Almost all premalignant and malignant cells of the cervix occur close to this transformational zone between one tissue and another. About 95 percent of cervix cancers derive from squamous (scaly) cells, and the remainder, which are called adenocancers ("adeno" means gland), from glandular cells. Clear cell cancer, which is common in daughters of women who took the drug DES during pregnancy, is a kind of adenocancer and may occur in the cervix, as well as more commonly in the vagina (see the section on vaginal cancer).

EARLY WARNINGS

Multiple studies show that actual cervix cancer is preceded by *in situ* cancer, and this, in turn, is frequently preceded by dysplasia. *In situ* cancer is the last stage prior to the occurrence of cancer. *In situ* means, literally, that the cancer is confined to its original site and has not penetrated the normal tissue. Dysplasia is a term describing cellular abnormalities that may precede *in situ* or true cancer. The changes are classified as mild, moderate, and severe to denote degrees of abnormality. These precancerous changes may reverse either with treatment or sometimes spontaneously. Dysplasia occurs most frequently in the twenty-to-twenty-nine-year-old age group; true cancer occurs most frequently after the age of forty. Women with dysplasia are at high risk for cancer *in situ,* and women with *in situ* are at high risk for invasive cervical cancer. One study found that 85 percent of women developing *in situ* or actual cancer had been previously diagnosed for dysplasia. However, the term dysplasia, and especially mild dysplasia, is so broad as to include almost anything abnormal found on a Pap smear including inflammation and infection, and some types of mild dysplasia are *not* associated with an increased risk of cervical cancer.

In view of the problems both of dysplasia classification and adequate patient follow-up, estimates of dysplasia progressing to *in situ* and *in situ* progressing to actual cancer have varied widely. In one report, among thirteen patients who had refused treatment for *in situ* cancer, ten progressed to actual cancer between one and fifteen years later. According to a different report, only a third of *in situ* patients progressed to actual cancer within a nine-year period. There is much variation in the speed of progression.

SYMPTOMS OF CERVIX CANCER

- None at the earliest stage.
- Thin, watery, blood-tinged vaginal discharge.
- Vaginal bleeding.

SYMPTOMS

Because there are *no* symptoms associated with dysplasia or *in situ,* regular Pap smears are essential in detection of early cervical changes. Probably the first symptom of early cancer is a thin, watery, blood-tinged vaginal discharge that may go unrecognized by the patient. If the cancer has penetrated deep enough to reach small blood vessels, then intermittent, painless, intermenstrual spotting or bleeding may occur. Or nothing more than spotting after intercourse or douching. As the malignancy enlarges, the bleeding episodes become heavier, more frequent, and of longer duration, and the patient may also experience what seems to be an increase in the amount and duration of her regular menstrual period. Eventually, the bleeding occurs daily. The bleeding is more likely to prompt early medical attention in a postmenopausal woman. Late symptoms include development of pain in the flank or leg, usually because of involvement of the sciatic nerves or even of the ureters, which carry urine from the kidney to the bladder. Finally, the extensive cancer may cause pain with urination, blood in the urine, bleeding from the rectum, or swelling of one or both legs.

WHO IS AT RISK?

Sexual Contact

Research has indicated that cervical cancer is generally related to patterns of sexual intercourse. Women with cervical cancer tend to have had first intercourse at an early age, multiple sexual partners, and have been the partner of men who have had multiple partners.

If her age at first sexual intercourse is between fifteen and seventeen, the woman's risk is tenfold that of a woman whose first intercourse occurred in her mid twenties. First intercourse between ages eighteen and twenty results in a sixfold risk; and between ages twenty-one and twenty-three, in a two-and-a-half-fold risk, all relative to those who had first intercourse in their mid twenties. If a woman has had one sexual partner during her lifetime, the relative risk of cervical cancer is minimal. If she has had two or three sexual partners, her risk is twofold that of the woman with only one sexual partner. If she has had more than nine sexual partners, her risk is 3.6 times that of a woman who has had only one mate. If she remains a virgin, her risk is less than one-tenth that of a woman with only one sexual partner.

Since early age at first intercourse and multiple sexual partners may occur in the same person, it is difficult to know which factor is the more important. If age at first intercourse is more important, it may be that some cancer-causing agent affects the developing cervix to a greater extent just after the onset of puberty but before the cervix has matured. On the other hand, if multiple sexual partners is the more important factor, the sexual transmission of some cancer-causing agent by the male is more likely. A greater number of partners would increase the chance of exposure to the carcinogen. Interestingly, *even if* the woman has only one sexual partner, if that partner has had many partners, the woman's risk increases. In this way, the risk of developing cancer of the cervix resembles the chance of contracting gonorrhea or syphilis.

In the past, the occurrence of cervical cancer in lower-class women has been higher than in women of the wealthier classes, with the poorest women having about five times the incidence of those in the wealthiest class. At least eight studies have noted this difference. Early age at first intercourse and multiple partners of either the women or her husband may explain the association between cervix cancer and the social factors. However, wealthier women may have been more likely to have the dysplasia and *in situ* conditions successfully reversed than were poorer women. Whatever the reason, this difference appears to have greatly diminished over the years, possibly because early age at first intercourse is now less influenced by socioeconomic class, or possibly because better health care is now available to the poor.

Women who have been married once have higher incidence rates than those who have never been married. Divorced and widowed women, and all those married more than once, have even higher rates. Women who were young at first marriage or who had either multiple marriages or multiple pregnancies are at higher risk. Women with more pregnancies tend to have married at a young age, however, and a greater number of pregnancies is not a risk factor once the age at first intercourse is taken into account. Cervical cancer has been found more frequently than would otherwise be expected in women who have had a sexually transmitted or venereal disease, especially syphilis. But this factor appears related to multiple sexual partners, and not to the cause of cancer.

Ten and twenty years ago incidence rates of cervical cancer were higher in urban areas than in rural, though the more recent data show that rural women now have greater rates of the disease. It appears that in city areas, women take greater advantage of Pap smears and doctor visits in general. More early abnormalities are thus found and treated before they can progress to cancer.

Herpes Virus and Cervical Cancer

Many investigators believe that previous herpes simplex type II infection—the common sexually transmitted disease—plays an important role in the development of cervix cancer. It has been proven that a herpes virus called the Epstein-Barr is related to human lymphoma and to cancer of the back of the nasal passages. Even though the sexually transmitted herpes virus does not produce cancers in animals, other herpes viruses do, including lymphoma in chickens, kidney cancer in frogs, and lymphoma and leukemia in rabbits, guinea pigs, monkeys, and gorillas. In these animal cancers, the DNA of the herpes virus is known to enter and transform the animal's normal genes, causing the cell to have cancerous characteristics, including uncontrolled growth and reproduction.

Circumstantial evidence suggests that herpes simplex type II virus is related to human cervix cancer: about 40 percent of severe dysplasia or *in situ* cells grown in the lab display evidence of this virus. However, if the patients from whom these cells were obtained had an ongoing herpes infection, the herpes virus may have been an innocent bystander. Still, herpes has been found to occur frequently in the same women who have dysplasia, *in situ* cells, and actual cancer. The average age for development of *in situ* cells is five to six years later than the average age for development of the herpes infection. Previous herpes infection is present about three times more often in patients with cervical cancer than in similar patients of the same age, socioeconomic class, etc. Twelve studies from different countries confirm this finding. When patients with herpes infections were followed for several years, the rate of developing cervix dysplasia was double and the rate of *in situ* changes was eight times the rate of a similar group of women who had never had herpes.

One limitation of the circumstantial evidence connecting herpes to cancer of the cervix is that some of it has been founded on antibody tests. Herpes simplex type I—a common nonsexual virus responsible for cold sores—is often not distinguishable from type II by antibody testing. Another criticism of the cervix cancer/herpes connection is that the virus grows preferentially in rapidly dividing cells, such as cancer cells. Accordingly, the virus might become associated with cervix cancer only after the cancer begins. The most convincing criticism is that cancer of the cervix and herpes may be associated only because of their mutual association with multiple sexual partners, early age at first intercourse, etc. Thus the question has yet to be resolved whether herpes is a factor causing cervix cancer or whether herpes simply tends to appear along with it for the reasons suggested.

Other Viruses

The papilloma virus, which causes genital warts, is transmitted primarily by sexual contact. The evidence that this virus is related to cervix cancer is even less than that for the herpes virus. The papilloma virus is found in only 1 to 3 percent of all women but is found in more than 20 percent of cervical biopsy specimens performed for abnormal Pap smears. Trichomoniasis, syphilis, and gonorrhea have sometimes been found together with cervical cancer, though these associations are believed to reflect life-style rather than causality.

Cigarette Smoking

Cigarette smoking has been found in numerous studies to be associated with cancer of the cervix. These studies were lightly dismissed on the assumption that there is a difference in the sexual behavior of smoking and nonsmoking teenagers. However, a 1983 study of young women with abnormal cells (dysplasia and *in situ*) found that a greater number smoked, even after age at first intercourse, multiple partners, and so on, were taken into account. Accordingly, cervix cancer may eventually be added to the list of tobacco-induced diseases.

Other Factors

Women who have had cancer of the vulva or vagina are at a slightly increased risk for cervical cancer, perhaps because these three areas have similar cells, embryologically derived from similar tissue. There is no increased tendency for cervical cancer in those who have had cancer of the uterus or ovaries, since the two organs do not contain similar tissue.

At one time it was believed that an uncircumcised male partner would increase one's chances of cervix cancer. For example, in India, where the Moslems practice circumcision, there is a low rate of cervical cancer; among the neighboring Hindus, who do not practice circumcision, there is a higher rate of cervical cancer. However, there are also other religious groups who do not practice circumcision but have low rates of this cancer. It is currently thought, therefore, that high or low rates are dependent on sexual practices deeply rooted in the religion and not on the usage of circumcision.

There are no known genetic factors predisposing a woman to cancer of the cervix and it does not tend to run in families. There have been several reported cases of cervix cancer development in women whose husbands were previously married to women with cervix cancer. There have also been several reported cases of cervix cancer in women whose husbands have had cancer of the penis. However, in both instances the number of patients involved is so small as to give rise to the association simply at random.

About 6 percent of cervix cancers are adenocancers, or adenocarcinomas. Although little is known of their specific causes, these cancers appear different from squamous cancers in that the patients are somewhat older, and multiple partners and early age at first intercourse do not seem to be factors.

A separate disease is the clear cell cancer of the cervix, usually occurring in the woman whose mother took DES while carrying her *in utero*. Although usually a vaginal cancer, clear cell cervix cancer can occur alone or in combination with vaginal cancer.

Prevention

CONTRACEPTIVE DEVICES. The birth control pill appears to have little influence on the development of cervix cancer. Barrier methods of contraception (i.e., rubbers and diaphragms) have been reported to protect against cervix cancer. This finding is believable inasmuch as barrier methods could protect the cervix from direct contact with semen and other external factors. However, because of the small numbers involved in these studies, other factors—such as age at first intercourse and number of sexual partners—could not be carefully analyzed. Therefore, it is not known whether barrier methods themselves protect against cervix cancer or if women with low risk for cervical cancer happen to choose the diaphragm or other barrier methods.

NUTRITION. Because there are pronounced nutritional differences between poorer and wealthier groups, vitamin deficiencies have also been studied. A relatively low vitamin C intake may predispose women to dysplasia, which is often the precursor of cervix cancer. One study asks whether the recommended minimum daily requirement for vitamin C, 60 mg, is enough for high-risk women. In that study, women with a daily intake of less than 30 mg of vitamin C had a sevenfold increase in dysplasia. This association appeared independent of such risk factors as low income, sexual frequency, or age at first sex. The physician conducting the study also noted that women with a daily intake of 10 mg of vitamin C had seventeen times the risk of women with a comparable sexual experience, etc., but who had a daily intake of 300 mg of vitamin C. The study suggested that high-risk women might decrease their chance of cervical cancer by increasing their intake of vitamin C to that level.

Another vitamin known to be important in maturation of lining, or epithelial, cells is vitamin A and similar compounds. Instead of increasing dietary dosages and thereby increasing blood levels, an experimental approach under study applies a vitamin A cream directly on the cervix. Two different studies are evaluating the results for women with dysplasia. Side effects include vaginal warmth and a stinging sensation. The results will not be ready until the late 1980s.

DETECTION AND DIAGNOSIS

The Pap Smear

The Pap test, in existence for thirty years, consists of the microscopic examination of stained cells taken from the cervix by scraping. The objective is to determine invisible precancerous and cancerous cellular changes. If any *visible* abnormality is present, it should be biopsied because a biopsy yields more cells than the Pap smear, allowing for better evaluation. As mentioned, cervix cancer is usually preceded by a series of changes. The changes range from mild to moderate to severe dysplasia and on to *in situ* cells, which are very similar to cancer cells, except that they have not penetrated into tissue as do true cancers. Remember that until true cancer develops, no symptoms whatsoever are associated with these changes. Blood-tinged discharge—usually the earliest symptom—occurs only when true cancer invades deeply enough into the tissue underneath.

Simplicity, acceptability, cost, and validity make the Pap smear one of the best cancer screening tests known. The test is simple and is quickly and easily performed by doctors, trained nurses, and paramedics. The fact that 75 percent of American women have had at least one test attests to its acceptability. The cost is that of a blood count. Its accuracy—finding abnormal cells if they exist—is 80 to 95 percent.

To get the best and most accurate Pap smear, a woman should not douche for at least two or three days before the test, since douching might wash away some abnormal cells. One should not use birth control foams or jellies for three days, or have vaginal intercourse for two days, before the appointment. The optimal time for the Pap smear is day fifteen to twenty of the menstrual cycle—just after ovulation; a Pap smear should not be done while a woman is menstruating. If abnormal bleeding is present, however, the Pap smear and pelvic exam should be performed anyway. Otherwise, the presence of a cervix or endometrial abnormality might go undetected while the patient waits. A common error is to delay the Pap test for two to three months because of intermittent or continuous spotting.

The usual procedure involves wiping the cervical canal with a cotton swab or aspirating the canal mucus; the outer area of the cervix is wiped with a flat wooden stick. Traditionally, the results have been reported in five classes: I, normal; II, atypical; III, suspicious; IV, carcinoma *in situ;* and V, cancer. Class II may be caused by infection or inflammation. Class III and beyond will require a follow-up biopsy with examination by the pathologist. Over the past five years, a new classification system, called CIN, has become more common than designation by Classes I to V. The initials stand for *c*ervix *i*ntraepithelial (within the outer lining) *n*eoplasia (literally, "new growth," in reference to abnormal cells). In contrast to the older, rigid classification, the CIN reporting acknowledges some overlap between the classes. The subdivisions of CIN are: (1) mild and mild to moderate dysplasia; (2) moderate and moderate to severe dysplasia; and (3) severe dysplasia and cancer. Roughly, CIN 1 includes Classes II and III; CIN 2, the more advanced part of Class III; CIN 3, classes IV and V.

How Often Should You Have a Pap Smear?

The American Cancer Society has recently made the following recommendations: low-risk women who have had negative Pap smears for two consecutive years can safely be tested thereafter once every three years. Two annual negative Pap smears are necessary since some studies show that a single Pap smear may falsely result in a negative report up to 20 percent of the time. This may result from such factors as menstruation at the time. Afterward, low-risk women should have a Pap smear at least once every three years until age sixty-five. Women at higher risk should be screened more frequently, as decided on an individual basis. A greater effort must be made to encourage high-risk women to have Pap smears, since women of highest risk are the least likely to have Pap tests.

Public health experts no longer recommend yearly screening of low-risk women because of the cost to the American medical system. A Pap test itself ranges from $8 to $25, assuming that the woman is already in the physician's or practitioner's office for other reasons. Otherwise, the test would cost between $25 and $40. In 1974, it was estimated that the cost of delivering, screening, and follow-up services to 80 percent of eligible women in the United States would be about $1 billion or 1 percent of annual United States health expenditures. On the other hand, the chance of finding abnormal cervix cells in low-risk women after two previous normal Pap smears is very low. For example, in first-time Pap smear screening of large numbers of women in Los Angeles, 500 out of 100,000 were found with dysplasia, 500 with *in situ* cells, and 150 with true or invasive cancer. Among women who had previously had a negative Pap smear one to seven years earlier, the rates were 240 out of 100,000 with dysplasia, 7 with *in situ,* and none with true cancer. This study suggests that the prevalence of significant cervix abnormalities, including cancer, is low among women who have recently had a normal Pap smear.

All statistical considerations aside, if you cannot be sure of being low risk, continue to have an annual Pap smear. Even if you are low risk, if the Pap smear gives you added peace of mind, that alone is reason to have one every year. The Pap smear's only drawbacks are the cost and inconvenience, and the benefits may save your life. If you are high risk for any of the previously listed reasons, a yearly Pap smear is advisable, even if repeatedly normal. And, needless to say, if any symptoms develop, a Pap smear should be performed at once.

TREATMENT OF MILD AND MODERATE DYSPLASIA

What is the next step if mild to moderate dysplasia has been discovered? An abnormal Pap smear is always repeated. Then, in order to confirm that no cells present are worse than those already known—and to discover where those cells are—the physician will carefully look for any visible abnormalities. The Schiller's test is performed to highlight any abnormal areas for biopsy. Schiller's solution is a weak iodine stain that is painted on the cervix; normal cells take up this temporary stain and turn darker. Any areas that remain light are abnormal and will be biopsied. In the case of mild dysplasia, if no abnormal areas are seen and a vaginitis is present, the woman will be treated for the vaginitis. A repeat Pap smear is necessary to make certain that the test becomes normal.

If dysplasia is persistent on a subsequent Pap smear, and no abnormality is visible, endocervical curettage and then colposcopy are usually performed. Endo (inside) cervical curettage consists of scraping out the canal cells—which cannot be seen—for microscopic analysis.

Colposcopy

A colposcopy follows the procedure of a usual pelvic examination. The speculum, an instrument used to separate the walls of the vagina and expose the cervix, is inserted as during a Pap smear. The cervix is swabbed with a solution of acetic acid, the major component of vinegar, to remove the mucus. The colposcope itself is a stereoscopic microscope that provides a brightly illuminated and magnified (ten to twenty times) three-dimensional image of the cervix, or vaginal walls. The colposcope instrument does not enter into the vagina at all. Although it takes some fifteen to twenty minutes longer, the exam feels no different than a pelvic exam. Different lenses are placed on the colposcope, which highlights abnormal areas. A photographic attachment on the side of the colposcope can record the appearance for subsequent comparison. Slight abnormalities—unseen by the naked eye—are graded on the basis of several characteristics. A satisfactory examination requires visualization of the cervix transformation zone, where the cells change character (glandular to squamous) and almost all cervical cancers begin. Colposcopy, then, is just the natural extension of what can be done with the naked eye. Its purpose is to find the area causing the abnormal cells found on the Pap smear. The area will then be biopsied to determine the degree of abnormality.

Colposcopy is not painful and does not affect fertility. Following colposcopy a slight brownish discharge may be noticed if biopsy was done because of the solution applied. Since this may be irritating to a partner during sexual intercourse, one should abstain for at least a day or two. Without biopsy, one can resume all activities, including sex, immediately after colposcopy.

Simple office biopsy directed by colposcopy is diagnostic in 99 percent of patients in whom colposcopy is satisfactory. Colposcopy is satisfactory only with visualization of the transformation zone where the cells change. In about 10 to 20 percent of women the transformation zone occurs higher up in the cervical canal, instead of on the outside, so that the zone cannot be visualized on colposcopy.

If colposcopy is inadequate, or unavailable in a particular community, and Pap smears are persistently abnormal, then it is necessary to perform a wider-reaching cone biopsy under general or spinal anesthesia.

Simple Versus Cone Biopsy

Simple cervix biopsy is done by an instrument with a sharp cup, measuring approximately an eighth of an inch in size, which takes a tiny amount of tissue. Biopsy is done without anesthesia because, unlike the skin in general, the cervix has a sparse nerve supply. The patient experiences nothing more than a tugging or pinching sensation. Afterward, there may be slight vaginal bleeding for a day or so.

A cone biopsy derives its name from the ice-cream cone–shaped specimen taken from the center of the cervix. The specimen includes the lower part of the canal and the zone of cell transformation. The

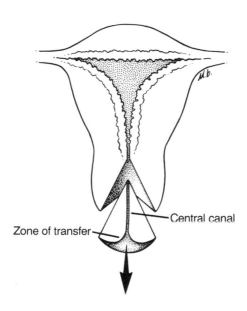

Cone biopsy

larger part of the cone is positioned toward the outside of the cervix and also includes any abnormalities visible on colposcopy. The cone biopsy is performed under general or spinal anesthesia and requires hospitalization for several days. While the cone biopsy provides a great deal of accuracy, early complications can include postoperative bleeding, making a return to the operating room necessary. Late complications include narrowing of the cervix canal in about 7 percent of the cases. Narrowing of the canal can interfere with exit of menstrual blood and with vaginal deliveries. Pregnancies after a cone biopsy have a slightly higher miscarriage rate. One is not permitted to have intercourse or put anything in the vagina for about six weeks following the surgery.

Before colposcopy, biopsy was largely by the cone technique. Cone biopsy is still frequently necessary for abnormal Pap smears where colposcopy is not available or fails to determine the area causing the abnormal Pap smear. As mentioned, since colposcopy often demonstrates the abnormal area, a simple office biopsy suffices. Nowadays, instead of diagnosis, cone biopsy is more often used for treatment of severe dysplasia, and of moderate dysplasia that persists after treatment, and occasionally for treatment of *in situ* changes.

Freezing—Cryotherapy or Cryosurgery

Cryotherapy—treatment by freezing—requires that the patient be positioned as for a Pap smear. Cryotherapy is best performed one week after a menstrual period, thereby precluding the possibility of an unknown pregnancy and providing maximal healing prior to the next menstrual period. Freezing gas, usually nitrous oxide, or carbon dioxide, from a tank by the patient's side, is applied for three minutes or so. Different applicator tips are available for abnormal areas of various sizes and distribution. Immediately following the procedure, one might experience cramps, similar to menstrual cramps, and some faintness. Afterward, most women have a heavy, watery discharge, sometimes blood-tinged, for two to four weeks. Tampons are not to be used, but one may wear sanitary pads. Mild cramps may continue for a few hours or a few days and may require pain pills for relief. Fever, pain worse than cramps, and true vaginal bleeding should be reported to the doctor. Douching and sexual intercourse are not advisable during the interval with heavy watery discharge.

Cryotherapy is a simple treatment performed in the doctor's office. It takes fifteen to twenty minutes, and often can be performed with an IUD in place. While the treatment presents minimal problems, the failure to permanently reverse the abnormality ranges from 4 to 50 percent, according to various reviews of the subject. The large range among studies is probably due to the lack of standardization of freezing techniques, different definitions of cure and failure, and difference in follow-up time. After cryotherapy, close follow-up with Pap smears is required every three months to detect abnormal cells that remain or recur.

Cryotherapy is effective in eliminating mild and moderate dysplasia. It has also been used experimentally on some patients with severe dysplasia. However, if the abnormal cells remain or return after cryotherapy, cone biopsy is often necessary. Also, if the abnormal area is large or extends into the cervical canal, a cone biopsy is advisable instead of cryotherapy. The cone biopsy performed for diagnosis is the same as that performed for therapy.

Thermocauterization, or destruction of cells by heat, an older but effective technique, is said to be more painful than cryosurgery. Laser therapy, presently experimental, is available in some areas, and may eventually take the place of cryotherapy.

Local treatment (cryotherapy, thermocautery, laser surgery) may be inappropriate in a variety of situations: if the total transformation zone is not visualized; if the scraping of the canal itself (endocervical curettage) reveals any cancer cells; if there is a lack of confirmation between Pap smear and colposcopy and/or biopsy; if any frank cancer is present, etc. Nevertheless, with abnormal Pap smears so common, the number of patients requiring and benefiting from local therapy is large.

TREATMENT OF SEVERE DYSPLASIA AND *IN SITU* CELLS

Severe dysplasia and *in situ* changes are usually treated by a cone procedure or a simple hysterectomy. The cone procedure for treatment of these changes is the same as that sometimes used to diagnose the abnormality. If a woman has completed childbearing, a simple hysterectomy is recommended as clearly the safer of the two procedures, since removal of all the cervix necessarily and definitively removes the abnormality. There is no chance of recurrence because there is no cervix. The ovaries may be safely left untouched. A cone procedure can remove the abnormal cells, and if the patient is willing to return faithfully for scheduled Pap smears and examination, she may be able to preserve the childbearing function. After the cone procedure, however, whether for diagnosis or for treatment of known abnormality, there is a slightly higher miscarriage rate.

Recently, a few centers have been performing cryotherapy for severe dysplasia on an experimental basis. However, it has not yet been determined that cryotherapy is effective enough for this degree of abnormality.

Staging

The extent of disease must be known as fully as possible to allow for the treatment—radiation, surgery, or both—appropriate to each individual. A careful physical and pelvic exam, as well as several additional tests, may be needed. The structures close to the cervix, which may be invaded by the cancer, such as the ureters, bladder, and rectum must also be evaluated. An intravenous pyelogram (IVP) is performed because of the proximity of the ureters (tubes carrying the urine from the kidneys to the bladder) to the sides of the cervix. In an IVP, dye is injected into the bloodstream and passes into the urine by way of the kidneys, thereby outlining the entire urinary tract. The IVP can also give some information about the bladder, although cystoscopy—actually viewing the inside of the bladder with a tiny scope—is often necessary. Since the bladder base is directly in front of, and the rectum is directly behind, the cervix, sigmoidoscopy—viewing the inside of the rectum with a scope—is also often performed.

Cervical cancer tends to spread early to the pelvic lymph nodes and to remain localized in the pelvis for a long time. However, it is important to determine whether more than the pelvic lymph nodes are affected by the cancer. If the lymph node involvement has progressed beyond the pelvis, surgery alone cannot be successful. In the past, lymphangiography has been important in determining spread in the pelvic and abdominal lymph nodes. In this test, X-ray dye is injected into the lymph vessels of the foot. The dye proceeds up the leg into the pelvic nodes and higher into the abdomen. If cancer is present within the lymph nodes, it should appear as an empty spot in the dye-filled lymph node. Because of the vagaries of lymphangiography and because a CT (computerized tomography) scan is more convenient to the patient, the newer test has replaced lymphangiography in many institutions. The CT scan is at least as reliable as lymphangiography. Occasionally, additional tests may also be recommended, when other areas of spread are suspected.

TREATMENT OF EARLY STAGES OF CERVIX CANCER

Treatment of early cervical cancer by surgery or radiation appears to produce equal results, though beyond the earliest stages, radiation is clearly the better treatment. There are significant but different complications from X-ray treatment or surgery.

Surgery

The surgical treatment is radical hysterectomy. The uterus is removed with the upper half of the vagina, in order to obtain a sufficient margin of uninvolved tissue. If an inadequate margin of upper vagina is removed, the invisible cancerous roots remain, only to re-appear and make their presence known within several months to a few years. Although ovarian hormones affect breast and endometrial cancer, they have no effect—good or bad—on cervical cancer. The ovaries, therefore, usually remain and younger women are able to go through menopause at the normal age.

In cervix cancers with the most superficial penetration, the frequency of lymph node spread is 1 percent. Therefore, it is not necessary to combine radical hysterectomy with removal of the pelvic lymph nodes. On the other hand, if the penetration of the cervix cancer is deeper, then both parts of the procedure are required, because of the higher statistical likelihood of cancerous lymph nodes. Sometimes, if the removed lymph nodes are cancerous, external X-ray therapy is given postoperatively. If such is planned, the retained ovaries may be surgically positioned higher in the abdomen during the radical hysterectomy. The ovaries remaining in the pelvis would otherwise be in the path of the X-ray beam and menopause would result from the beam's effect.

There are significant complications to a radical hysterectomy. Of course, any four- to six-hour procedure involving moderate blood loss entails more risk to the patient who is either elderly or who has serious preexisting diseases. But in addition, there are complications specific to radical hysterectomy and pelvic lymph node removal. Because the pelvic lymph nodes lie close to the ureters, 1 to 5 percent of women experience uncontrollable postoperative urine leakage (from the vagina) for a time. This distressing complication is treated with catheter drainage of the bladder and frequent changes of sanitary pads. Fortunately, it almost always heals by itself within a matter of weeks. The removal of tissue around the bladder tends to weaken the bladder's muscular tone, causing inability to empty the bladder completely. Drainage by a urinary catheter for two or three weeks postoperatively is also the treatment for this complication. A minor problem involves lymph fluid collections in the pelvis after removal of the pelvic lymph nodes. Left untreated, the fluid usually reabsorbs; otherwise, it must be drained with a needle.

Because of the veins involved, any operation in the pelvis has the possibility of producing a blood clot. If the blood clot, called an embolus, breaks loose from the pelvic vein, it could go to the lungs, causing a pulmonary embolus, which is a serious complication. Pulmonary embolus can occur after any operation, but is more common after pelvic operations, including routine hysterectomies, cesarean sections, and bladder procedures. Early postoperative leg exercise should decrease the chance of vein clots.

The total removal of the uterus through a vaginal incision has been widely practiced in some areas of Europe. However, almost all American gynecologic oncologists strongly believe that the operation should be performed through an abdominal incision, owing to the improved visual exposure. The upper portion of the pelvis, including the ovaries and the adjacent structures of the lower abdomen, are not visualized through a vaginal incision. The standard abdominal incision allows removal both of the cancer with a wide margin and any adjacent structures necessary.

Radiation

X rays can be used effectively at early stages of cervical cancer and is the treatment of choice for all later stages. Depending upon the exact location and extent of disease at time of diagnosis (i.e., the stage), either internal or external radiation or both are used.

Internal radiation involves inserting an applicator designed to stay securely on the cervix. The applicator has holes that keep the radioactive sources in place and is usually fitted in the operating room under general anesthesia, with the radioactive sources, in turn, fitted to the secured applicator when the patient has been returned to her room. The cancer-destructive rays of the radioactive isotopes, though traveling only short distances, have considerable power, so that it is necessary to keep the radioactive applicator in place for only a day or so for the necessary amount of treatment. Enemas are given before placement and a catheter is used to drain the bladder, allowing the patient to maintain strict bedrest during the treatment.

The applications may be repeated a second time if extra radiation is necessary. Such short-distance radioactive isotope treatment will not affect organs at a greater distance, such as the ovaries, which should continue to function normally. However, the area being irradiated—the cervix and upper vagina—do gradually scar, harden, and shrink. While the bladder base is occasionally affected, it is only after several months or years that, for a small percentage of patients, a decreased bladder capacity might result in frequent trips to the bathroom. The hardening and dryness of the vagina caused by radiation treatment can be problematic for the younger, sexually active woman. Since surgery avoids this problem, it is often chosen by younger women and older women alike who are in good physical shape, even though complications particular to surgery are more numerous than those particular to radiation.

If pelvic lymph nodes are found to contain cancer cells at the time of radical hysterectomy, *external X-ray treatment* is often necessary to treat invisible cells that may be left behind. As mentioned, pelvic X-ray treatment damages the ovaries, usually inducing early menopause.

Even though the uppermost portion is removed, women do not usually notice a decreased vaginal length during sexual intercourse, since the remaining normal vagina will stretch sufficiently. If it does not, certain positions in sexual intercourse, such as keeping the thighs together, simulate greater vaginal length.

Treatment of Cervix Cancer During Pregnancy

The diagnostic procedures of Pap smear, colposcopy, and office biopsy can be used on pregnant women with no danger; a cone biopsy, however, does pose a significant risk of miscarriage. If the patient desires the pregnancy but also requires treatment for cervical cancer, the baby can be delivered near term by cesarean section, with a radical hysterectomy performed in the same operation. Such a procedure is longer and more difficult than a standard radical hysterectomy, since both the pelvic blood supply and the uterus itself are so much larger than in the nonpregnant woman. Nevertheless, such operations occur often enough, since women who have avoided routine Pap smears may be found to have cervical cancer only on their first obstetric visit. A radical hysterectomy can be performed early in the pregnancy despite the presence of the fetus, if an abortion is desired.

TREATMENT OF LATER STAGE CANCERS

As mentioned, radiation, and not surgery, is the treatment for all stages beyond the earliest. Surgery simply cannot remove all the cancer and therefore is not used. In most of these cases, both internal radioactive sources and external beam treatment are used. Sometimes, because of the location and greater amount of cancer, only external X-ray treatment is used.

The larger the extent of cancerous area to be treated, the greater and the more frequent the complications. Still, only 5 to 10 percent of treated patients have serious bladder and/or rectal problems, sometimes consisting of abnormal connections between the bladder and vagina or rectum and vagina. Most will experience sexual dysfunction from vaginal narrowing, dryness, and radiation-induced menopause.

Chemotherapy

Cancer-killing drugs are most often used if the pelvic cancer recurs after maximum radiation or if the cancer has spread from the pelvis. Administration of chemotherapy can be a problem in this instance because the pelvic blood supply, through which the drug would travel, has been decreased by the scarring process following surgery or X-ray therapy. Therefore, delivery of chemotherapy drugs to the pelvic cancer site is diminished. Also, kidney function may be decreased because of ureter obstruction from the cancer, such that some of the effective drugs, if excreted by the kidney, are unusable. In addition, the bone marrow reserve for blood cell production may have been decreased with the extensive prior irradiation and may cause the patient to be prone to infection. Keep in mind, also, that chemotherapy drugs injure bone marrow, although this is usually temporary. In spite of these difficulties, chemotherapy is an active area of research, and progress is being made. Cisplatin or CPDD (Platinol) is one of the most effective current drugs, though possible side effects include kidney damage, ringing in the ears, and tingling of the fingertips and toes at the higher doses.

Results and Recurrence

The overall five-year survival and cure rate for cervical cancer is 57 percent. It is slightly higher in whites (59 percent) than in blacks (48 percent), a difference mostly reflecting the greater extent of disease in blacks at the time of diagnosis. When only localized disease is considered, survival rates, averaging 77 percent, are similar for both whites and blacks.

The most common site of recurrence is in the pelvis itself, close to the original cancer. Almost half of those who die of cervix cancer have the disease still localized, although extensively present, in their pelvis. This is not the case in most other cancers, such as breast or colon cancer, where almost no one dies from malignancy that remains localized.

A far-reaching operation called pelvic exenteration can cure some patients with a localized recurrence. This massive operation removes the uterus, fallopian tubes and ovaries, rectum, bladder, ends of the ureters, and all the lymph nodes in the area. Basically, all the usual pelvic structures that may be involved with cancer are removed. The intestines, which are loose and movable, refill the space. Since the natural exits for the fluid and solid waste are no longer present, the two substances must exit separately through the abdominal wall and are collected by bags. The most commonly used method for detouring the urine is the same as that used after removal of the bladder for bladder cancer, and calls for joining the ureters to an isolated loop of bowel and bringing one end of the loop to the skin surface, where it is covered by a bag. The loop remains disconnected from the rest of the bowel, thereby preventing mixture with the stool and consequent infection. The urine flows to the outside of the body through this system. (Both this skin exit and the one used for solid waste are called stomas.) The result requires a constant bag appliance, since urine travels into the bag constantly. Because urine is thin and watery and tends to leak, a stoma therapist must teach the appliance fitting technique. Even though one must empty the bag every four hours or so during the day, the appliance itself is left in place for five to seven days. One showers or bathes with it on.

Usually on the other side of the abdomen, a permanent colostomy is fashioned in the same manner as that after an operation for rectal cancer. Since most of the colon remains, the waste material will be solid and somewhat formed, as it would be under normal circumstances before the operation. Accordingly, the colostomy can be trained to function only once a day, usually with a morning enema given in the bathroom. For the rest of the day, the stoma can be covered by a large Band-Aid.

The Endometrium (Uterus)

The uterus, an organ measuring three inches by two inches by one inch, touches the bladder with its front side and the rectum with the back. In its spherical shape and tapered proportions, the uterus resembles a pear. The bulk of the body, the larger spherical part of the pear, consists mostly of muscle surrounding a small cavity. The smaller, stem end of the pear corresponds to the cervix or the uterine neck. The cervix, which is the outlet for the uterus, projects into and is totally surrounded by the vagina. It can easily be seen and felt during the pelvic exam. The function of the uterus is to aid in the transpor-

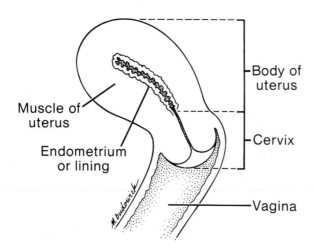

Side view of uterus

tation of sperm, to hold the fertilized egg, and to protect the fetus and help it develop through the nine months of pregnancy.

The inside lining of the uterus, or endometrium, undergoes cyclical monthly changes, including shedding itself as menstrual blood. This lining is the origin for endometrial cancer, also commonly, but somewhat incorrectly, called uterine cancer. Cancer may also arise separately in the cervix. The two cancers, cervical and endometrial, tend to occur in entirely different groups of women. Cervical cancer occurs in younger women, who have had early intercourse, and perhaps an early pregnancy. Endometrial cancer is more common in older women who have never been pregnant.

Approximately one in every thirty women in the United States, 3.3 percent, will develop endometrial cancer. In 1980, there were 38,000 new cases, but only 3,200 deaths resulting from the disease. Accordingly, it is a common, but not particularly aggressive cancer. Endometrial cancer is rare before age forty, and then becomes increasingly common with age until the early sixties, after which the rate decreases somewhat.

Endometrial cancer is third in the list of most common cancers in women, while ranking ninth as a cause of female cancer deaths. The death rate from this cancer declined from the 1950s through the 1970s, owing, most probably, to early detection and treatment. The incidence of this cancer remained unchanged until the late 1960s, when the frequency of endometrial cancer began to rise. Fortunately, the increase has been in the early and easy-to-treat varieties.

SYMPTOMS OF ENDOMETRIAL CANCER

- Vaginal spotting or bleeding.

SYMPTOMS

The main symptom for all endometrial cancers is vaginal bleeding. In fact, bleeding, or even spotting, either between menstrual periods or after menopause, is just about the only symptom. Other symptoms are caused by spread to other organs, a rare occurrence. However, while vaginal bleeding is a symptom of endometrial cancer, it can also result from other causes, such as vaginitis, fibroid tumors, hormone imbalance, and polyps in the cervix or uterus. Even vigorous sexual intercourse immediately preceding one's normal menstrual period can cause bleeding or spotting. In postmenopausal women who receive estrogen (for relief of menopausal symptoms and for conditions such as osteoporosis), bleeding may be due to the estrogen itself. Nevertheless, *any* nonmenstrual vaginal bleeding requires an explanation.

WHO IS AT RISK?

Various factors have been associated with increased risk of endometrial cancer. Many of these risk factors are associated with *excess* estrogen, whether produced in the body or taken by mouth. There is, however, no known increase in endometrial cancer caused by use of oral contraceptives, probably because they contain only a small amount of hormone. Occasionally, a given woman's estrogen level, though within the range of normal, is too high, because it is not adequately balanced by the opposite hormone, progesterone. Such a woman may be predisposed to endometrial cancer. While there is no genetic predisposition to this cancer, it may occur in the same family, because the related women have the same high-risk factors.

Fat

One factor that predisposes a woman to endometrial cancer is excess weight. Very heavy women are at particularly high risk, while the risk among slightly overweight women is only slightly higher than the risk in normal weight or underweight women. In fact, women fifty pounds overweight are ten times more likely than women of normal weight to develop endometrial cancer. Even though the disease most often occurs in older women, very obese women are among the youngest women with this cancer.

Why does excess fat predispose a woman to endometrial cancer? An enzyme found in the fat converts androstenedione, a normal hormone made by the adrenal gland, into estrone, a type of estrogen. Accordingly, obese women have higher estrogen levels circulating in the blood than do thin women. In fact, excess estrogen may be what prevents many obese women from ovulating and being able to conceive.

Infertility and Childlessness

There is general agreement among researchers that women who have never been pregnant are at higher risk for endometrial cancer than women who have, and that the more pregnancies a woman has had, the lower her risk. Although only 24 percent of postmenopausal women in the United States have never been pregnant, over 50 percent of women with endometrial cancer have never been pregnant. Many childless women are infertile, and infertility can be due, among other causes, to either high or normal estrogen levels without sufficient progesterone.

Women with the Stein-Leventhal syndrome (polycystic ovaries) are generally infertile. In this syndrome, ovulation does not take place, and even though the woman bleeds intermittently, she does not have true menstrual periods. The level of circulating estrogen tends to be high. Also, a condition such as polycystic ovaries tends to be accompanied by high levels of adrenal hormone, which can be converted into estrogen. Women who do not ovulate regularly and have long intervals between menstrual bleeding may be at risk of endometrial cancer due to the body's failure to shed the uterine lining regularly. The fact that the endometrium remains in place for long intervals without the normal shedding and replacement may somehow predispose it to malignancy.

Postmenopausal Estrogen Replacement

Researchers in thirteen leading studies have found an increased risk of endometrial cancer among women who undergo postmenopausal estrogen replacement. The elevation of risk has generally ranged from twofold to eightfold. The longer the medicine has been used, the higher the risk. Women who have taken the medication for eleven to fourteen years are twenty-five times more likely to develop uterine cancer than similar women who have never used estrogens. However, after fifteen years of use, there appears to be no further increase in risk. The increase is dose-related, so that a woman taking a higher dose is at greater risk. Fortunately, when use of postmenopausal estrogen stops, the risk decreases rapidly.

After menopause, the endometrium, deprived of estrogen, becomes thinner. Estrogen replacements stimulate the endometrial cells, which proliferate and become thicker. In the past, medical experts prescribed a regimen of estrogen replacement taken daily, 365 days a year. The overgrown endometrial lining, remaining in place for long periods, may promote the development of malignant cells. Since this information has become available, women who require postmenopausal estrogen are given the smallest daily dose that relieves symptoms and are advised to take it for only three out of every four weeks.

Estrogen users who are diagnosed with endometrial cancer tend to be younger than those who have not used estrogen. Fortunately, most of the cancers found in women taking postmenopausal estrogens are discovered at the earliest stage, when the malignancy is confined to the endometrium itself. One study found that the five-year survival or cure rate in estrogen users with adequate treatment was 94 percent.

While estrogen is associated with increased risk of endometrial cancer, postmenopausal hormone replacements that contain both estrogen and progesterone may not be. In Finland, postmenopausal replacement includes both hormones, and the Finnish women who take the medication do not have as high a rate as women in the United States who take just the estrogen. However, since Finnish women may be protected by some other factor, such as lack of obesity, the difference in hormone replacement treatment may not be responsible. More research is required in this area.

Estrogen replacement seems to increase the risk of endometrial cancer more for thin than for fat women. On the other hand, estrogen therapy may only *seem* to be more cancer-causing in thin women, since the risk is naturally so high in fat women that the additional risk from estrogen replacement has little effect.

Animal experimentation shows that prolonged administration of oral estrogens causes cancer in the endometrium of various species, such as rabbits, mice, and rats, and that progesterone may be protective. Also, administration by constant daily dosage rather than daily dosage by cycles (three weeks on, four weeks off) is more cancer-causing in animals.

It has been suggested that because estrogen replacement induces bleeding, it alerts the physician that endometrial cancer is present—in other words, that postmenopausal estrogen replacement results in the discovery of many early cancers, but does not cause it. However, most doctors maintain that estrogens have much to do with the actual cause. As mentioned previously, the incidence of endometrial cancer began to rise in the late sixties and early seventies. The greatest increase was among women aged fifty to fifty-nine and was most marked in women of higher socioeconomic class, who are the greatest users of postmenopausal estrogens. Within the United States, the rate for whites is about twice as high as that for blacks, which may reflect greater use of postmenopausal estrogen by white women.

In summary, the longer the estrogen use, the greater the risk. Stopping postmenopausal estrogen decreases the risk. Perhaps most importantly, the human findings parallel the results of animal investigations.

Miscellaneous Factors

Many studies have reported a higher risk of endometrial cancer among diabetics. In turn, it is at present unclear to what extent the combination of diabetes and endometrial cancer is attributed to obesity. Hypertension has also, to some degree, been associated with an increased risk of endometrial cancer, but this, too, may be related to obesity. A late menopause—past age fifty-five—increases the risk of endometrial cancer somewhat. This is thought to be caused by the additional time such women experience the premenopausal levels of estrogens. A common condition, called endometriosis, in which the endometrial lining can be found outside the uterus, has no relation to endometrial cancer.

DETECTION AND DIAGNOSIS

The Pap smear, so effective in detecting cervical cancer, samples only the cells of the cervix, and is not useful in detecting endometrial cancer. When patients with confirmed endometrial cancer were evaluated, only 40 percent had abnormal cells showing on a Pap smear. In those cases, the malignant cells were passing through the outlet of the cervix at the time of the Pap smear.

The use of uterine aspiration, although a more complex procedure than the Pap smear, can be performed in the doctor's office. In this procedure, a very thin tube is inserted through the opening in the cervix into the endometrial cavity, and a small amount of tissue is scraped from the lining. This test, however, detects only some endometrial cancers, not all. Another office procedure is the "jet" irrigation and washing out of endometrial cells for analysis.

A pelvic exam is very important for evaluating the extent of the disease. The uppermost vagina, a common place for spread of endometrial cancer, can be seen with the aid of the standard speculum instrument. The size, shape, and mobility of the uterus is determined in that part of the pelvic exam where the doctor inserts one hand in the vagina and places the other on top of the abdomen. In addition, the fallopian tubes and ovaries, both common areas for spread, can also be evaluated.

The D and C (dilatation and curettage) procedure is useful for obtaining tissue not only to confirm malignancy, but also to determine the differentiation of the cancerous cells—how well or poorly they resemble normal cells. In a D and C, the opening to the cervix is stretched and enlarged, while the patient is under anesthesia, to permit passage of the curette instrument into the uterine cavity. Following dilatation, first the lining of the cervical canal and then the lining of the body of the uterus is scraped with a simple, semisharp loop, and tissue samples are taken. The specimens from the two parts of the uterus are collected and examined separately, since it is then possible to determine whether the endometrial cancer has also grown downward to involve the cervix. During the procedure, a "sounding," or measurement, of the inside length of the uterine cavity is taken. The inside length of a normal postmenopausal uterus is three to four centimeters—less than two inches. Any greater length usually results from the cancer's enlarging the uterus.

Staging

Once endometrial cancer has been diagnosed, a course of treatment is decided upon, with the treatment depending on the extent of the disease at the time of diagnosis. Determining the extent of disease is called staging. Some factors in staging, such as the increased size of the uterus, are evaluated in physical exam or during the D and C. Other factors become apparent only after the uterus has been removed, when the involvement of the fallopian tubes, ovaries, and/or pelvic lymph nodes is evaluated. Perhaps because endometrial cancer, more than other cancers, causes obvious symptoms at an early stage, the malignancy is localized to the lining of the uterus in about 75 percent of the cases.

A chest X ray and intravenous pyelogram (IVP)—an X-ray dye test that outlines the kidneys, bladder, and the ureters connecting them—are usually done before treatment. Occasionally, it may be necessary to examine the interior of the bladder and rectum by means of a cystoscope and sigmoidoscope, since both organs are immediately adjacent to the uterus and likely sites for spread. The differentiation of the cancer cells is also important in predicting an individual patient's course of treatment. Patients with well-differentiated cancer—cancer with cells more closely resembling normal cells—have significantly greater survival rate than those with the same extent of disease and poorly differentiated cancer cells.

TREATMENT

Surgery

Assuming the patient is in otherwise good health and able to undergo anesthesia, surgical removal of the uterus, fallopian tubes, and ovaries through an abdominal incision is almost always the treatment for endometrial cancer. Technically, the term "hysterectomy" means only the removal of the uterus. It does not include removal of ovaries or tubes, which are removed as part of an endometrial cancer operation. However, the term is often used vaguely and many women who have undergone hysterectomies do not know precisely what was removed.

It is generally agreed that patients diagnosed at the earliest stage have a greater than 90 percent prospect of being cured by surgery and will need no additional therapy, such as radiation. On the other hand, if, at the time of the hysterectomy, the cancer is found to have spread into the lymph nodes, tubes, or ovaries, then postoperative radiation therapy is usually recommended. Chemotherapy is used in the treatment of endometrial cancer only in those rare cases when the cancer has spread to distant sites.

The kind of hysterectomy necessary for endometrial cancer is rarely more extensive than that performed for fibroids or other benign diseases and is usually much less extensive than that for cervical cancer. Since radiation is effective for prevention of recurrence in endometrial cancer, it is not necessary to remove the uppermost vagina to prevent recurrence, as in the case of cervical cancer. Therefore, after surgery the vagina will be as extended and close to its normal shape as possible.

Removal of the uterus alone does not normally affect sexual desire or activity. On the other hand, removal of the ovaries in premenopausal women will result in immediate menopause, regardless of age. The patient will probably then begin to notice a lack of lubrication during sexual intercourse just as if she were postmenopausal. The dryness results from lack of the hormone estrogen and can be corrected either with a vaginal lubricant or with an estrogen cream. Since some estrogen is absorbed into the bloodstream through the vagina, the individual must have no contraindication to estrogens, such as endometrial cancer which has spread, or breast cancer.

Some women, especially younger women, will not notice dryness or other changes following the removal of their ovaries. In such cases, the adrenal glands produce hormones that, to a greater or lesser degree, take the place of the missing estrogen. If the woman is already postmenopausal, removing the uterus and ovaries for endometrial cancer, or for any other reason, should produce no change in vaginal condition and sexual functioning.

A vertical incision, from at least the navel to the pubic bone, is recommended for hysterectomy in endometrial cancer, since it provides a good view of the pelvic structures and can be extended upward above the navel if necessary. In some hysterectomies, the low transverse or horizontal incision, almost in the pubic hairline, is often employed for a greater cosmetic effect. However, the surgeon who selects this "bikini" incision must be prepared to close it and make a vertical incision if necessary to allow for better surgery or pelvic lymph node removal. In other words, the incision must not be permitted to limit the operation. In the presence of an enlarged uterus, of cancerous extension to the cervix, or of an enlarged ovary, the maximum operating area can be obtained only through a vertical midline incision. Sometimes, depending on the patient's size and build, the remaining abdominal organs cannot be seen with the cosmetic bikini incision.

If use of a small abdominal incision means a more difficult operation, one can imagine how much harder it is to perform a hysterectomy by means of vaginal access. This approach is often used for nonmalignant diseases—it decreases the complications, the length of time spent in the hospital, and the general difficulty in recovering from the operation. In a woman whose uterus is normally drooping downward through the vagina, because of weak pelvic support, this kind of hysterectomy is easier to perform. For obese patients also, a vaginal incision is often used, because the obesity does not interfere as it does with an abdominal incision. Given these reasons, some doctors advocate removal of the uterus, fallopian tubes, and ovaries through the vagina (no abdominal incision) even though the surgeon is unable to visualize any spread of the disease and it is more difficult to remove an enlarged uterus, or bulky tubes and ovaries this way. Still, a vaginal hysterectomy is sometimes the recommended approach. For example, it might be performed as a compromise between an abdominal-approach hysterectomy and no surgery for an obese patient with severe medical problems.

Radiation

Radiation is effective in preventing recurrence in the vagina for almost all patients. The vaginal recurrence, which can appear within a year or two, usually results from microscopic extensions unseen at the time of surgery and therefore untreated. Since only 25 to 33 percent of patients with recurrence in the vagina can be cured, it would seem reasonable to supplement hysterectomy with radiation therapy for those patients at risk. However, there is no clear-cut agreement on how radiation and surgery are best combined. *Preoperative external X-ray treatment* by cobalt or similar X-ray machines has the advantage of encompassing the whole pelvis, decreasing the chance of cancer cells being shed and implanting into the vagina or elsewhere at the time of the operation. Such treatment can also kill cancer cells in the pelvic lymph nodes, which may escape during the surgical procedure. One disadvantage of the preoperative approach, though, is the delay required, in most instances, to allow the patient to recover from the acute effects of radiation before undergoing surgery. This may involve four to six weeks of X-ray treatment, followed by two to six weeks of rest. Because radiation causes changes in the tissue treated, another disadvantage of preoperative radiation therapy is the difficulty of determining the depth of the cancer's invasion into the muscle of the uterus; in other words, since the uterine tissue has been changed by the radiation, accurate staging becomes more difficult.

However, *postoperative external X-ray* treatment allows the extent of the patient's disease to be determined before the administration of any further treatment. Knowing the true extent of the disease from accurate surgical observation should allow for greater accuracy in matching the extent of treatment to the extent of the disease. It has not been clearly demonstrated that one X-ray treatment program is superior to another for all patients.

Another use of X ray concerns *preoperative internal radioactive sources*. These are placed into a device that, in turn, has been inserted directly into the uterus, usually under general anesthesia. The sources are kept in place for several hours. The high-dose, short-distance radiation affects virtually only the uterus, and this is some-thing of a disadvantage because the pelvic lymph nodes remain un-treated. However, external X rays can be used in the standard way postoperatively. Preoperative X-ray treatment by insertion of radio-active sources allows the surgery to be performed within several days with no increase in complications. Moreover, the extent of cancer in-vasion is easier to assess because there has been little time for radia-tion-induced changes in the tissue. In some instances, the radioactive sources are used twice, some weeks apart, followed by another rest of several weeks before surgery.

For early cancers, the best course is probably to remove the uterus, fallopian tubes, and ovaries; to biopsy the pelvic lymph nodes; and to sample the abdominal fluid. Postoperative X-ray therapy may then be administered in the few cases where cancer has unexpectedly reached into the muscle of the uterus or has spread to the lymph nodes, tubes, or ovaries. Additional therapy is necessary because such spread may not be limited to the organ removed.

Chemotherapy and Hormonotherapy

Chemotherapy for endometrial cancer has the usual consider-able side effects, which can include nausea, vomiting, hair loss, fa-tigue, and weakness. It is used for those few patients whose disease has spread outside of the pelvic organs. In spite of its rather severe side effects, doxorubicin hydrochloride (Adriamycin) is often used be-cause it is effective in shrinking tumors.

Hormonal therapy, if the cancer responds well to it, is preferable to chemotherapy, since administration of progesterone derivatives—hydroxyprogesterone (Delalutin) or medroxyprogesterone (Depo-Provera or Provera)—has virtually no side effects. It is used mainly for can-cers that cannot be successfully handled with radiation therapy.

The Placenta (Trophoblastic Disease)

The placenta, which nourishes the fetus until birth, develops from the fetal tissue after conception; like the fetus itself, it is composed of genes from both the mother and father. During the first half of pregnancy, the placenta grows at the same rate as the fetus. By the time the baby is born, the placenta is a structure about seven to eight inches in di-ameter and one inch thick, weighing a pound or more. Among other functions, the placenta routes all blood and oxygen to the infant and manufactures the hormone, human chorionic gonadotropin (HCG), which is partly responsible for maintaining the pregnancy. Moles, or benign tumors, of the placenta occur at the approximate rate of 1 per 2,000 live births. Trophoblastic cancers—choriocarcinomas—occur in about 1 out of every 40,000 pregnancies, whether abortions, ectopic, or normal deliveries. Trophoblastic is another word for placenta-derived and is related to terms indicating nourishment and growth.

The benign tumors and cancers arising from the placenta are unique because they are not composed solely of a woman's own genes and chromosomes: half the genetic material of each tumor cell is that of the woman; the other half that of her mate. Every other benign tumor or cancer is composed exclusively of cells arising from the person's own genes. Just as skin grafts from another person are rejected and organ transplant patients must be intensively medicated to prevent rejection, normal or cancerous cells placed into another person's body are immediately recognized as foreign by the immune system, which starts the destruction of such cells. Thus, benign tumors and cancers arising from the placenta are partially foreign, which may assist the body's immune system in recognizing and rejecting them.

Still, before intensive chemotherapy techniques were developed, more than half of patients with trophoblastic cancers died within the first year, as did virtually 100 percent of patients whose disease had spread to distant organs. Perhaps because the placenta itself grows so rapidly, this cancer is also one of the fastest to enlarge and spread. Yet cancer of the placenta, choriocarcinoma, was the first cancer to be cured by chemotherapy alone, without surgery or radiation therapy. And a woman may retain her reproductive organs and produce healthy offspring after treatment for, and cure of, this disease.

SYMPTOMS OF TROPHOBLASTIC DISEASE

- Vaginal bleeding during pregnancy.
- Abnormal uterine growth during pregnancy.
- Passing tissue vaginally.

EARLY WARNING OF HCG

Human chorionic gonadotropin (HCG) is produced by the normal placenta, and pregnancy tests are based on finding this substance in the urine or blood. All tumors of the placenta, whether benign or malignant, produce this hormone. Unless she is pregnant or has a placenta-derived tumor—or, rarely, an unusual germ cell tumor of the ovary—no woman should have any amount of this hormone in the blood. As such, HCG is really the perfect tumor marker. It is found in only two cases: when a tumor is present or when a woman is pregnant.

Moreover, the level of HCG exactly parallels the amount of placenta-derived cells in the body: a high level signifies a large amount of tumor. This level will fall in response to chemotherapy and disappear when the patient is cured. Even such sophisticated tests as CT (computerized tomography) scans come nowhere near finding such small amounts of disease as can be found with a simple blood test. If tumor markers of this quality existed for other cancers, detection and treatment would become greatly simplified and more effective.

The frequency of *benign* tumors (moles) arising from the placenta is 1 per 2,000 hospital deliveries in North America and Western Europe and rises to 1 per 200 in Southeast Asian countries. In both areas of the world, older women are at higher risk. The risk per pregnancy is three times higher in women over forty than in women twenty to twenty-four. The risk is believed to increase twenty-fold for pregnancies after age forty-five. Although poor socio-economic conditions leading to poor nutrition might be responsible in Asian countries, there is no association with poor nutrition and/or low income in this hemisphere. Only about 2 percent of moles become cancers. On the other hand, of all such cancers, half arise from and are preceded by, a molar pregnancy. There is no evidence supporting a familial predisposition for benign tumors or cancers originating from the placenta.

EARLY WARNING AND TREATMENT OF MOLAR PREGNANCY

Molar pregnancy is a benign condition in which abnormal placenta tissue grows in the uterus after the union of egg and sperm. Over 95 percent of the time there is no recognizable fetal tissue and the mole is the sole product of the fertilized egg. Because the patient has all the symptoms of a normal pregnancy, including an enlarging uterus, diagnosis of a molar pregnancy is usually made only when the molar tissue, which appears as uniform maroon fleshy material, is passed.

Of women with molar pregnancies, 89 percent experience bleeding (in three-quarters of women this occurs before the fourth month of pregnancy), 14 percent vomiting, and 10 percent pain. The nausea and vomiting that accompany a molar pregnancy are difficult to separate from the same symptoms found during a normal pregnancy. One indication of a molar pregnancy is that uterine size is often not what one would expect from calculating the date of the last menstrual period: half of such patients have a uterus size greater by at least one month's growth than one would expect by reckoning from the date of conception. The diagnosis is often suspected around the fourth month because of the symptoms, abnormal uterus growth, and inability to hear the fetal heart sounds with a stethoscope. Detection is facilitated by ultrasound, which shows the honeycomb pattern of a typical mole.

Treatment of a molar pregnancy involves simple evacuation of the contents of the uterus by suction or vacuum curettage. (Precisely the same procedure is used to induce a therapeutic abortion during the first trimester of pregnancy.) Under anesthesia, a vacuum tube is inserted into the uterus and simply draws the molar tissue forth. After a molar pregnancy, a woman should have a physical with pelvic and rectal exam every two weeks for at least two months and certainly until the uterus has returned to normal size and vaginal bleeding has stopped.

About 15 to 20 percent of benign moles cannot be cured by simple vacuum suction, because they have grown into the wall of the uterus. It will not be apparent at the time of the suction curettage which women require further treatment, though subsequent blood test analysis for HCG will usually make the determination. When all placenta-derived tissue is absent, the level of HCG will return to normal. But for those women in whom the abnormal tissue has grown into the uterine wall, the HCG level remains high. These women will require either a hysterectomy or simple chemotherapy. Women who have finished their childbearing may choose to undergo a hysterectomy (ovaries may remain). Women who wish to have (more) children will opt for chemotherapy so as to retain the uterus.

While only 2 to 5 percent of moles turn cancerous, such cancer usually spreads rapidly to other parts of the body. For patients at high risk either for cancer spread to distant organs or for mole growth into the uterine wall, preventive chemotherapy is usually administered. The high-risk category includes such factors as a very high HCG level, a large amount of molar tissue, the woman's age (greater than forty years), and toxemia, usually evidenced by high blood pressure, during the molar pregnancy. In other words, before either of the two consequences has time to develop, preventive chemotherapy, usually with actinomycin D (dactinomycin), is started.

ORIGINS AND TREATMENT OF CANCER OF THE PLACENTA (CHORIOCARCINOMA)

About half the patients with cancer of the placenta and distant spread will not have had a previous molar pregnancy. They have had a previous pregnancy with a normal delivery, an ectopic pregnancy, a spontaneous miscarriage, or a therapeutic abortion. Choriocarcinoma is, however, a thousand times more likely after a molar pregnancy than after any other kind of pregnancy. The uterus usually does not return to its normal small size and may continue to bleed. As opposed to the tissue of a molar pregnancy, the tissue of an actual cancer is rarely passed spontaneously. Diagnosis is, therefore, more difficult to make until there are symptoms in distant organs that will alert the physician to draw the HCG blood test. In fact, some medical authorities have suggested that a woman who has previously had any kind of pregnancy followed by cancer spread from an unknown site should have an HCG blood test to eliminate the possibility of this rare cancer.

Patients with choriocarcinoma can currently be cured even when the disease is widely spread from the uterus. About 90 percent will not only be cured by chemotherapy, but will also be able to avoid surgery and keep their uterus, allowing for further childbearing. In fact, multiple pregnancies of treated women have resulted in completely normal offspring.

Chemotherapy involves either single or multiple drugs. Since multiple drugs give rise to more complications, patients are classified as to low- or high-risk and receive either single or multiple drugs on that basis. Low-risk categories usually include patients with spread to the pelvic organs, including the vagina, and to the lungs. High-risk categories include those with spread to the gastrointestinal tract, kidney, liver, and brain. If the patient is not cured with the single drug, even if she was in a low-risk category, she will then be treated with multiple drugs, while still retaining a high chance of cure. In fact, the cure rate now approaches 100 percent in patients with disease that has not yet spread and 85 to 90 percent in patients with disease spread to distant organs. Although spread to the brain and liver are most difficult to treat, they are still amenable to cure. Accordingly, treatment at a specialized center for this rare disease is crucial.

The drugs are given as rapidly and as closely together as can be tolerated, so as to eliminate the greatest number of cancer cells before they become resistant to the drug. The chemotherapy is so intense as to make its administration difficult and dangerous. The drug-induced damage to normal organs, such as the bone marrow, is not evident until five to ten days after the end of drug administration. Accordingly, a chemotherapist must reduce the drug's dosage if greater damage of normal tissue is suspected, but must avoid compromising the patient's chance of cure by too great a reduction. For these reasons, patients should be treated only in centers where they can receive expert attention. The facility must include not only a large enough laboratory for careful monitoring, but also such sophisticated intensive care unit treatments as platelet and white blood cell transfusion and absolute isolation.

The Ovaries and the Fallopian Tubes

In a premenopausal woman the ovaries are white, oval structures measuring about one and a half inches by one inch, with surface folds and ridges. After menopause, they shrink in size to measure less than one by one-half inch. Located low in the pelvis, about two to three inches on either side of the upper uterus, the ovaries are partially wrapped by the fallopian tubes.

The ovaries have two primary functions: to secrete the female sex hormones, estrogen and progesterone, and to contain eggs, one of which matures and is released with every menstrual cycle. The hormones produced by the ovaries help the vagina maintain a normal thick surface with appropriate secretions; the hormones also regulate ovu-

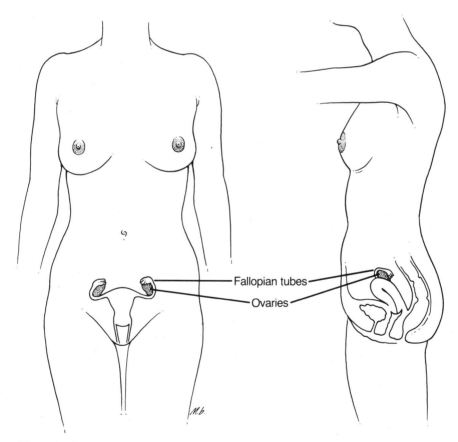

Fallopian tubes
Ovaries

Front and side views of fallopian tubes and ovaries

lation, the menstrual cycle in general, and pregnancy to some extent, among other functions. Ovulation occurs about two weeks before the menstrual period when the matured egg, stimulated by pituitary hormones, bursts forth from the surface of the ovary and into the nearby fallopian tube.

Ovarian cancer ranks fourth behind breast, lung, and colon cancer as a cause of cancer death among American women. About 19,000 new cases of ovarian cancer are diagnosed yearly among women in the United States, and it has been estimated that about one out of every seventy-two women will develop ovarian cancer. Ovarian cancer accounts for a quarter of all gynecological malignancies but causes about half of all gynecologic cancer deaths. It is thus the leading cause of death from gynecologic cancers in the United States, surpassing by a small margin the death rate from cervical and endometrial cancer combined.

The kind of ovarian cancer responsible for 90 percent of occurrences is rare among women in their twenties and thirties, but starting around the age of forty, the incidence increases with each decade.

Ovarian cancer refers to a group of malignancies that arise from the widely different kinds of cells present in the ovaries. The varied cells bear little relationship to one another. The three main types of cells are the epithelium, or lining and surface, cells; the stromal, or supporting, cells; and the germ, or egg-related, cells. Ninety percent of ovarian cancer arises from the epithelium, so that the great majority is of one common type. The other two are uncommon, and have different biological characteristics.

It is rare for cancers to produce hormones. Therefore, cancers arising in the stromal, or supporting, tissue are of particular interest, although they comprise less than 5 percent of ovarian cancers, because they may produce not only estrogen, but sometimes also androgens, the male hormone. There are no symptoms of excess estrogen if the woman is premenopausal. In the postmenopausal woman, an estrogen-secreting cancer would produce the same signs as that of estrogen replacement pills, such as postmenopausal uterine bleeding. If the cancer is producing male hormones, virilizing may occur—manifested by an increase in facial and body hair and deepening of the voice.

Germ cell cancers, those arising from cells related to the egg itself, occur mainly in children and young adults. They are rare even in these age groups and represent overall less than 2 percent of all childhood malignancies. Germ cell cancers are heavy tumors that often grow on their own stalks. Twisting of this kind of tumor on its stalk occurs as a complication in 10 to 20 percent of cases, causing acute abdominal pain and discovery of the cancer. Germ cell cancers are unusual because they may manufacture one or two abnormal hormones.

These hormones, human chorionic gonadotropin (HCG) and alpha feto protein (AFP), are normally found in the blood only during pregnancy or with rare diseases. If the cancer produces these hormones, analysis of the blood is a convenient way to check for the cancer's recurrence.

A small percentage of cancers discovered in the ovaries is metastatic, that is, it has spread from the site of origin in the stomach or breast, to name two likely cancer sources.

SYMPTOMS OF OVARIAN CANCER

- A sensation of heaviness, fullness, or expansion in the low pelvic area, usually without much pain.
- An enlarging belly, probably first noted by an increase in belt size.
- An enlarged ovary found incidentally during a pelvic exam.
- Frequent urination and/or constipation (caused by an ovarian mass pressing on the nearby structures).

SYMPTOMS

Because the ovary is in a hidden location, an ovarian cancer does not usually produce any clues as to its presence until it is at an advanced stage. Whether benign or malignant, an ovarian mass can grow quite large—while producing minimal symptoms—or not at all. It will push the loose, flexible small bowel and colon aside and fill the space. If anything, it may cause a sensation of fullness or heaviness in the pelvic area. Because of its location in the body, an ovarian mass may also press upon the bladder, causing frequent urination in small amounts, or upon the lower colon or rectum, causing constipation. There is usually no vaginal bleeding, as with early endometrial cancer, and the Pap smear, which can detect the earliest cervical cancer, almost never reveals an ovarian cancer. Consequently, more than 70 percent of ovarian cancers will have spread outside the pelvis by the time of diagnosis.

The most common symptom of ovarian cancer, and the one that leads about 45 percent of patients to seek medical attention, is an enlarging abdomen. Swelling may result from the size of the mass or, more likely, from the accumulation of fluid in the abdominal cavity, which contains shed cancer cells. Specifically, the patient may notice an increase in her belt size or a bulge in the mid and lower abdomen. Abdominal swelling due to fluid may also be the result of nonmalignant causes, ranging from severe liver disease to heart failure. The second most common symptom of ovarian cancer, causing its discovery in a third of the cases, is pelvic pain or pressure, which is caused by the tumor pressing on other structures. Third, an actual pelvic mass is found during physical exam in 9 percent of patients. Fibroids, common benign tumors of the uterus, can grow quite large and sometimes produce pelvic pressure and frequent urination. Fibroids, however, do not produce abdominal fluid. Four percent of women with ovarian cancer had unexplained weight loss, while 10 percent had a variety of miscellaneous symptoms leading to diagnosis.

WHO IS AT RISK?

International comparisons of incidence and death rates from ovarian cancer must be interpreted cautiously because of differences in classification, diagnosis, treatment facilities, and completeness of reporting. Nonetheless, a comparison can be useful in providing indications of cause. There appears to be an increase in the incidence of ovarian cancer in many economically privileged areas of the world as compared to the so-called developing countries. However, Japan, with its high standard of living and low rate of ovarian cancer, is an exception. Japanese immigrants to the United States and their first generation offspring have a greater occurrence of ovarian cancer than Japanese living in Japan. The second generation of Japanese immigrants to the United States has almost the same incidence of ovarian cancer as the United States population. The Japanese second generation rate is sixfold the rate of Japanese living in Japan. This suggests the influence of some local environmental factor, whether in the life-style or diet in the new community. Although the link has not yet been proven, many researchers suspect diet and diet-related hormonal changes. In fact, the populations of countries with high fat consumption generally exhibit higher incidences of ovarian cancer, as well as breast, endometrial, and colorectal cancer.

Women with any one of the three hormone-related cancers—breast, ovarian, and endometrial—have a slight predisposition to developing one of the others. Although thought unrelated to hormones, the susceptibility to cancer of the colon and rectum is also associated with these three. All four cancers are generally found in countries with an excessive fat, and especially animal fat, consumption.

Several studies have shown that women who have never been pregnant are one-and-a-half to three times more likely to develop ovarian cancer than women who have been pregnant. Furthermore, among women who have been pregnant, those with ovarian cancer had fewer pregnancies. Various theories have been advanced to explain the relationship between ovarian cancer and pregnancy, and it may be possible that some unidentified hormonal abnormality may predispose women both to ovarian cancer and partial or complete infertility.

High risk has been shown to exist among married but never-pregnant women.

According to another theory, pregnancy itself is protective, and ovarian cancer is promoted by the pituitary hormones, which govern the menstrual cycle and ovulation. Pregnancy not only interrupts the menstruation but also results in a lower blood level of pituitary hormone for the nine months. No association has been observed with irregular menstrual periods, length of ovarian cycle, heavy menstrual flow, duration of flow, or painful periods.

Another theory concerns ovulation. During ovulation, the release of the egg causes a rupture of the surface of the ovary. The frequency of this minor "injury" and/or the subsequent repair process may contribute to the development of cancer. This theory is supported by observations that such cancers are rare in animals that ovulate infrequently, such as the dog, but common in animals that ovulate frequently, such as the domestic egg-laying hen. Ovarian cancer is the most common cancer in that animal species. Furthermore, hens that are forced to lay more eggs than average (by artificially shortening their day) develop more ovarian cancers. Conversely, hens that experience fewer ovulations, and lay fewer eggs, develop fewer ovarian cancers. This strengthens the theory that the greater the number of ovulations in a woman's life, the greater the risk of ovarian cancer. The theory is compatible with the fact that ovarian cancer is highest among women who have never been pregnant and moderate among those who have been pregnant only once or twice.

To take this theory a step further, a decreased incidence of ovarian cancer has been observed in women who have used birth control pills and may be the result of the suppression of ovulation during the years of the pill's use. Since 1960, when the pill was widely promoted in the United States, more than 40 million American women have used oral contraceptives. After more than two decades of widespread pill use, a study by the National Cancer Institute shows that women who have taken the pill long-term are half as likely as other women to develop cancer of the ovary. The protective effect was seen in women who started taking the pill some fifteen years ago and who took it for eleven years or longer. As the only contraceptive method to suppress ovulation, the pill might decrease ovarian cancer for precisely that reason. However, this is not definite. The pill itself may not protect against ovarian cancer; women who take the pill may share an unknown factor that protects them.

The pill also reduces the levels of pituitary hormones, which control ovulation. In some laboratory animals, a high level of pituitary hormones by itself will cause ovarian cancer; some researchers believe that it is not ovulation but the increased pituitary hormones that are related to human ovarian cancer.

Miscellaneous Risk Factors

Though X rays have been shown to produce ovarian cancer in mice, the cancer is not of the same cell type as occurs in 90 percent of humans. Of the survivors of radiation from the atomic bomb blast, there were only slightly more cases of ovarian cancer than would have occurred in Japanese women under normal circumstances. Nevertheless, it is wise to shield the ovaries if possible while X-raying other organs.

Standard postmenopausal estrogen replacement therapy does not appear to increase the risk of ovarian cancer. However, when diethylstilbestrol (DES) was given in addition to the standard estrogen replacement, there was an increase in the rate of ovarian cancer. It has been proven that DES produces ovarian cancer in dogs.

In a very small percentage of cases, there may be a familial factor. I believe, however, that the mother/daughter cases more likely result from another factor common to the two patients, such as a similar pregnancy history. A study from Denmark found thirty ovarian cancer patients had identical twins; in only one case did the other twin develop the disease. Thus, no genetic factor has been suggested by this study.

DETECTION AND DIAGNOSIS

When symptoms of ovarian cancer occur, the disease has usually reached an advanced stage. The only simple way to diagnose ovarian cancer before symptoms appear is the pelvic exam. As mentioned, the Pap smear is not effective in finding ovarian cancer. With one or two fingers in the vagina, and the other hand on top of the abdomen, the doctor can compress the ovaries between the two hands and evaluate their size. Obviously, the ability to feel a small amount of enlargement is more accurate in thinner women. In women with thick abdominal walls, it is more difficult not only to detect an enlargement, but also to distinguish it from a fibroid of the adjacent uterus. Such benign tumors are common; one out of five women between the ages of thirty and forty-five eventually has fibroids to some degree.

If a questionable ovarian enlargement is felt, the next step is a pelvic ultrasound or a pelvic CT scan. Both tests are effective and may be able to differentiate enlarged ovaries from fibroid tumors with certainty, allowing the patient to avoid surgery.

Laparoscopy

Often, a laparoscopy, a procedure more minor than a surgical exploration, can be performed to visualize both ovaries and uterus. With the patient under general anesthesia, a lighted telescopic tube the size of a thick ballpoint pen is inserted through a one-inch incision, usually just below the navel. Before the insertion, the abdomen is filled with carbon dioxide gas to separate the abdominal wall and protect the organs inside. The gas is let out through the laparoscope at the end of the procedure.

Through this scope, the surgeon can view the surface of the abdominal organs. Often the procedure is performed with the patient's legs up in stirrups in the pelvic exam position. With a surgical assistant manipulating the uterus slightly through the vagina—as is done during a routine pelvic exam—the complete surface of the uterus, as well as both ovaries and tubes, can usually be viewed through the scope. Distinguishing between normal and enlarged ovaries or between fibroid tumors of the uterus and enlarged ovaries is usually successful. This procedure, needless to say, is important in evaluating many kinds of pelvic conditions. Of course, a previous operation or tubal infection may interfere with the viewing and even preclude attempting the procedure. Usually, only a one-day hospital stay is needed for this "Band-Aid" surgery.

TREATMENT

Ovarian cancer almost always requires an exploratory operation for diagnosis as well as for treatment. The exception may occasionally occur when the patient has definite spread outside the abdomen (e.g., to the lungs, which can be determined by a chest X ray). As in most other cancers, the treatment required and the prognosis depend upon two factors: the stage, the extent of the cancer at time of diagnosis, and the differentiation, the degree of abnormality of the cells.

Most cancers—such as breast, colon, and lung—are spread to distant organs through the lymph and/or blood vessel system. But an ovarian cancer often spreads by malignant cells that are shed from its surface. These cells float in the abdomen and are capable of implanting themselves on any surface. This occurs particularly in the pelvis, though spread to the underside of the diaphragm is not unknown. The other method of spread is through the lymphatic vessels (as with other cancers), into the pelvic lymph node system, and from there into the abdominal lymph nodes. Spread through the blood vessel system rarely occurs. The malignant fluid common in ovarian cancer is produced in two ways: the implanted malignant cells on the abdominal wall surfaces may "weep" fluid, or the lymphatic vessels may become obstructed with cancer cells, resulting in the lymph fluid collecting in the abdominal cavity.

Staging

It is absolutely essential to "stage" ovarian cancer accurately so that the amount of treatment administered corresponds to the stage. An adequate staging operation includes removal of the normal small amount of abdominal fluid (not more than a few ounces) and a "washing" of the surfaces of the pelvis and abdomen. This results in samples adequate for the detection of microscopic amounts of malignant cells, should they exist. The surgeon will examine all lining surfaces of the abdomen, including the undersurface of the diaphragm. All abnormal-appearing lymph nodes should be biopsied, while certain other lymph nodes, known as frequent sites of spread, are always biopsied even if they appear normal. The omentum, a fatty pad of tissue lying in front of the intestines, provides a large surface and is probably the most frequent site of spread. It is removed if abnormal and biopsied if uninvolved. Sometimes it is removed even if it appears normal. The surgeon will also remove the ovaries and any site to which disease has spread, as long as the patient's safety is not compromised. If ovarian cancer had spread to the bowel surface, for instance, requiring a colostomy, the surgeon may decide, depending on the individual circumstances, that so extensive a procedure would give little benefit.

Such operations to stage and treat ovarian cancer are substantial, and therefore require a relatively long vertical incision—particularly necessary for viewing the organs of the upper abdomen. Unfortunately, a cosmetic-appearing, short, horizontal scar above the pubic hairline, the so-called bikini incision, is totally inadequate. This small an incision limits visualization, and a mistake may be made in underestimating the stage or extent of spread.

As mentioned, the extent of spread determines extent of treatment. In one study, about 30 percent of patients who had undergone their original surgery at various nonspecialized hospitals were found to have more extensive disease when examined in a thorough staging operation at a cancer center. Without the second operation to accurately determine stage, such patients would have undergone less treatment, with the diminished likelihood of cure.

TREATMENT

The treatment of ovarian cancer has undergone great improvements in the past several years. There is an emphasis on removing as much cancer as possible, even if the cancer has spread widely throughout the abdomen. Such aggressive surgery is recommended because highly effective chemotherapy drugs exist for this cancer—more so than almost all other solid cancers. Therefore, if only small bits of cancer are left, even if throughout the abdomen, effective chemotherapy drugs can destroy them. Radiation therapy is also more effective with smaller cancers. The results include long survival and even cure for some cancers that have already spread. This operation, relatively specific to ovarian cancer, is called debulking or cytoreductive surgery.

Initial Surgery and "Second-Look" Surgery

In localized ovarian cancer, initial surgery is performed on all visible disease with a standard removal of the ovaries, fallopian tubes, and uterus. However, without additional therapy, about half such patients have a recurrence: the remaining microscopic deposits of cancer cells grow and eventually cause symptoms in the ensuing months and years. Therefore, additional treatment in the form of chemotherapy, radiation therapy, or both is recommended for almost all patients. The only exceptions would be patients with cancers in the earliest stage and those where the malignant cells are considered well differentiated (i.e., more like normal cells).

In the case of the initial surgery on advanced cancer, if the multiple cancer lumps can be surgically removed so that all remaining deposits are smaller than a half inch, chemotherapy will often produce long-term survival, as well as some cures. A recent study notes that half of such patients live over three years and about 20 percent live past five years and may be considered cured.

Determining whether chemotherapy has achieved the aim of destroying all cancer cells is accomplished by "second-look" surgery—either laparoscopy or a complete exploratory operation. Such procedures are necessary because the same lack of symptoms characteristic of the original cancer makes recurrence difficult to detect. Small amounts of disease spread on the abdominal linings cannot usually be detected by nonoperative means. Almost half the patients who have normal physical exams and normal ultrasound and CT scans after chemotherapy still have cancer—a fact that can be diagnosed by a second-look operation.

Some physicians use laparoscopy to check for obvious recurrence. However, laparoscopy might not be effective for some patients because of adhesions from the previous operation. In these kinds of patients, the possibility of damage to the bowel necessitates a formal operation. Open exploratory surgery and examination of all the organs must be performed to be absolutely sure there is no cancer. If no cancer is found during a full exploratory operation, chemotherapy drugs can usually be stopped. If cancer is found, it might be debulked again, and different and more aggressive chemotherapy drugs might be administered.

Chemotherapy

Virtually all drugs used in chemotherapy have side effects. Most cause bone marrow depression, with a consequent decrease in the number of platelets, which are important in clotting blood, and white blood cells, which are important in fighting infection. Sometimes there is also a decrease in the number of red blood cells over the long term. With hexamethylmelamine and cisplatin or CPDD (Platinol), nausea and vomiting are most common. Some drugs, such as doxorubicin hydrochloride (Adriamycin), act quickly to produce a temporary hairlessness. Methotrexate (Folex or Mexate) and 5-FU or fluorouracil give rise to short-term sores inside the mouth and throat. Cisplatin is excreted in the urine and may precipitate into crystals in the kidneys, causing permanent damage unless enough urine volume dilutes it. Cyclophosphamide (Cytoxan) may cause bloody urine by injuring the bladder lining unless it, too, is diluted. Hexamethylmelamine and cisplatin can occasionally give rise to a permanent condition of numb fingertips. Other complications can include liver damage by methotrexate, cardiac damage with Adriamycin, and lung damage with bleomycin sulfate (Blenoxane). Lastly, a long-term complication of chemotherapy drugs, particularly the class called alkylating agents, is the increased risk of leukemia decades later, especially if X-ray treatment has also been given. In other words, bone marrow–related cancers may be caused by virtue of the drug's profound effect on dividing cells in the bone marrow.

Usually a minimum of three different drugs are used at the same time. Since the drugs act in different ways, cancer cells that respond to one drug might not respond as well to another. Thus the maximum cancer cell destruction is obtained by combinations instead of single agents.

Because of their high toxicity and multiple side effects, it is especially important that the drugs be administered and the patients cared for only by chemotherapists experienced in ovarian cancer. It is always important to weigh the probable drug side effects against the possible benefits in each case. In ovarian cancer, with such effective chemotherapy available, the benefits often outweigh the side effects.

Research trials at cancer centers have included injection of chemotherapy drugs through tiny indwelling catheters throughout the abdomen. The catheter, the size of a long, flexible needle, can be placed at the time of surgery or inserted later without an operation. Because ovarian cancer often remains confined to the abdomen, this type of chemotherapy administration allows higher concentrations of a drug to be maintained in direct contact with the tumor for longer periods. Toxic symptoms to the rest of the body may also be lower than with intravenous administration. However, sometimes adhesions do not allow uniform drug delivery throughout the abdomen; if such is the case, this experimental method will not be useful.

One method of identifying effective chemotherapy drugs is the stem cell assay, in which cancer cell samples are taken from an individual, then cultured in the laboratory. This allows various drugs to be tested on an individual's cancer without treating the patient. If a given chemotherapy drug does not kill cancer cells in the test tube, it will not do so in the patient. Therefore, useless drugs, with their serious side effects, can be avoided. Since only a few places in the country perform this test, and because the test requires several weeks, the stem cell assay is usually performed only when standard chemotherapy drugs fail. One of the main drawbacks to this procedure is the fact that an individual's cancer might not grow in the laboratory; only about half do.

Radiation

Before the development of successful chemotherapy drugs, X-ray therapy was used widely and with moderate success as a preventive measure after surgical removal of the maximum possible cancer. Standard external X-ray treatment to the whole abdomen and pelvis is necessary because of the pattern of spread in this kind of cancer. Unfortunately, however, such sensitive organs as the liver and kidneys cannot tolerate as much X-ray energy as is required to kill cancer cells effectively. Lead shields are a mixed help: They protect both the organs and any cancer cells on them from the effects of radiation.

External X-ray treatments to the whole abdomen damage the bone marrow, which requires four to six months to recover. About 30 percent of the body's bone marrow—which produces the blood cells—is in the irradiated abdominal area. The remaining 70 percent will usually suffice, though a problem may arise if intensive chemotherapy, which also affects the bone marrow and its blood-producing elements, is required. In addition, whole abdomen radiation will produce temporary intestinal problems, such as diarrhea and cramping, and may produce permanent intestinal problems, such as adhesions and obstruction.

Intraoperative infusion into the abdomen of fluid containing radioactive isotopes was used widely as a preventive measure a decade or two ago. Its popularity decreased because other methods, particularly chemotherapy, proved as effective, while not exposing the operating team to any radiation. Some centers still use the intraoperative infusion. The isotope bathes all abdominal surfaces without penetrating and harming organs. The commonest radioactive element used is phosphorus 32, which emits short-distance radiation. The maximum effective range is two to four millimeters (i.e., about one-quarter inch). The main complications, as with external X-ray treatment, are intestinal adhesions and small bowel obstructions. In part, this may be caused by uneven distribution of fluid within the abdominal cavity.

CANCER OF THE FALLOPIAN TUBES

This cancer is rare, with fewer than 1,000 cases each year in the United States. It is also puzzling as regards the causes of gynecologic cancers. The endometrium originates in the embryo from the same tissue as the fallopian tubes and is a frequent area of malignancy. Why should structures with the similar embryologic background and cell type have different responses to cancer-causing agents? Part of the answer may be that cancers seem to develop more often in organs that undergo extreme physiological change than in those that are more dormant. The body of the uterus has monthly cyclical changes accompanied by significant hormonal and cellular alterations. The cervix is exposed to many external factors with intercourse and contraception. Both parts of the uterus are greatly changed by pregnancy and delivery. The fallopian tubes are more protected in that they are less involved in these events. The symptoms, age of onset, means of detection, and treatment of fallopian tube and ovarian cancer are similar.

Lung Cancer

The lungs are spongy organs filling most of the chest cavity. They enfold the other organs in the middle of the chest, including the heart, large blood vessels, and the esophagus, or food passageway. The main airway, or trachea, passes through the neck, then divides into two branches, or bronchi, for the two lungs. While it is very common for cancer to originate in the bronchi, it is less common for it to develop in the main airway. The smaller airways, also common sites for cancer, are formed by the continuing division, or branching, of the bronchi, which continue to divide until the terminal airways are formed. Each of these smallest airways, which measure about 1/1,000 of an inch across, terminates in an air-exchange unit called an alveolus. Within these alveoli, numbering some 3 million, oxygen from the inhaled air is exchanged for carbon dioxide, the waste gas produced by the body.

Cancer of the lung is among the most common and fatal of cancers, responsible for 5 percent of all deaths in the United States. The incidence of lung cancer rises with age. It is responsible for the greatest number of cancer deaths in men in the United States. In women, lung cancer has also been increasing yearly and within a few years, it will cause even more deaths than breast cancer (the current leading cause of female cancer death).

Were the term "epidemic" applied to any cancer, it would most

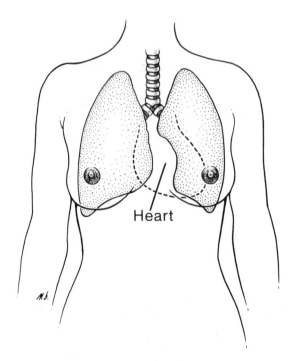

Heart

Shaded areas indicate lungs

accurately describe lung cancer. The disease was rarely found prior to the twentieth century; however, as automation and the development of cigarette manufacturing machines made mass production of inexpensive cigarettes possible, cigarette smoking became popular, and the rate of lung cancer began to rise. In 1920, there were only two cases of lung cancer diagnosed for 100,000 people. The incidence now exceeds 65 cases per 100,000. Because the cure rate is very low, not even reaching 10 percent, the number of lung cancer deaths closely parallels lung cancer incidence. In 1950, there were 18,300 deaths from lung cancer in the United States. About 110,000 were projected for 1983—a sixfold increase in just thirty years. This increase reflects the smoking habits of Americans. The occurrence of lung cancer in most countries parallels rates of consumption of cigarettes or other tobacco products that are inhaled.

While the male-to-female ratio in lung cancer rates long reflected the fact that more men smoked than women, the incidence of lung cancer in women has risen more than 400 percent since 1950 as women have begun to smoke in greater numbers. In the 1960s, the ratio of men to women developing lung cancer was ten to one; now that women's smoking habits more closely approximate those of men, the ratio approaches three to one. Yearly increases in lung cancer deaths show no signs of leveling off, and rates for women show greater yearly percentage increases than rates for men. Although women dying of lung cancer presently number less than men, a similar death rate is likely as the number of women who have smoked two to three decades begins to equal that of men who have smoked as long.

All lung cancers tend to arise from the lining of the airways. While it commonly arises in the lining of the larger airways, the lining of the smallest airways, leading immediately into the alveoli, can also develop cancer. Animal experimentation has demonstrated that repeated injury to the airways initiates mild abnormalities in the cells, which progress, over the years, to become malignant.

Physicians recognize four common types of lung cancer, differentiating them by the cell of the cancer's origin: squamous (scaly cell) cancer; adenocancer (arising from the glands); large cell cancer; and oat cell, or small cell, cancer. Together, these forms of cancer account for 95 percent of lung cancer. With the exception of oat, or small, cell cancer, which requires a different kind of treatment, the other three are almost the same as far as the lay person is concerned.

Squamous cancer, which comprises 30 to 40 percent of lung cancer cases, tends to occur in the larger airways, to grow more slowly, and to spread more within the lung (including its lymph nodes) than to distant sites. The oat cell type grows most rapidly and spreads earliest to other organs. The other two types—adenocancer and large cell cancer—spread less quickly than oat cell. The pattern of growth, while of some importance to treatment, makes little difference to cure rates. The lungs are richly supplied with blood and lymph vessels, and this may be responsible for a quicker spread than occurs with cancers arising in other organs, even when the cancer is quite small.

SYMPTOMS OF LUNG CANCER

- For smokers, any change in cough (sound, intensity, time spent coughing, and so on) or any change in mucus, or sputum, production (such as amount, thickness, color).
- For nonsmokers, any cough that lasts more than ten days.
- Chest pain or ache.
- Any amount of coughed-up blood.
- Wheezing.

SYMPTOMS

Coughing is the most common symptom reported at the time of diagnosis of lung cancer. Over 90 percent of lung cancer patients are smokers who most often notice a change in the character of their chronic cough. Any change at all—the sound or intensity of the cough, the time spent coughing, etc.—in such high-risk persons is reason to seek a chest X ray. Sometimes it is not the cough but the characteristics—amount, thickness, color—of mucus, or sputum, produced that have changed and should be reported. Nonsmokers should seek a physician's evaluation for any cough that lasts more than ten days, even if the cough itself is the only symptom.

Chest pain is the second most common symptom reported by lung cancer patients. It may occur as a persistent ache, unrelated to a cough, and is usually experienced on the same side as the cancer. It is possible, though less common, for the pain to feel like a slight stab that comes with each breath.

Blood-streaked mucus, or sputum, while often thought of in connection with lung cancer, is not usually the first symptom—and if other symptoms are present one should certainly not wait for its appearance before consulting a doctor. However, the smallest amount of blood in the sputum, even if it occurs but once as flecks, should be reported to the doctor. More than half of all lung cancer patients eventually cough up blood, although it is rarely the first symptom.

Wheezing may be an early symptom. A wheeze sounds like a musical note or whistle during inhalation or exhalation. It can be caused by the growing cancer's interference with the airway flow. The whistling noise occurs as the air passes the narrowed part.

Sometimes lung cancer is first noticed during a hospitalization for pneumonia, since the cancer in the airway can cause pneumonia by obstructing the airflow to the lung beyond. Without air exchange, the lung beyond the cancer fills with fluid and becomes infected, thus producing symptoms and resulting in a chest X-ray image of routine pneumonia. After the pneumonia passes, it may be possible to visualize the cancer. Unfortunately, lung cancer is sometimes not suspected until pneumonia has reoccurred several times.

Because of the rapid nature of its spread, lung cancer often produces no symptoms arising from the lung. The individual's first symptoms arise from the cancer's spread to other organs, and include yellowing of the skin, or jaundice, from spread to the liver; fits, or seizures, from spread to the brain; weakness; weight loss; and so on. Symptoms of spread within the lung itself include hoarseness caused by the involvement of the nerves controlling the larynx, or voice box; shortness of breath because of the involvement of the nerves controlling the diaphragm; swelling of the head, neck, and arms caused by compression of the veins from those areas; and difficulty in swallowing because of involvement of the esophagus, the food passageway connecting the throat and the stomach.

Though lung cancer most often appears as a single spot on a chest X ray, only about 40 percent of solitary spots, according to a Mayo Clinic report, are due to a malignancy of any kind. Lung cancer accounts for only 30 percent. Scars of an old fungus infection—usually not even noticed as a disease while ongoing—account for almost half of these single spots, called infectious granuloma. Ten percent are due to a cancer that has spread to the lungs from a starting point in a different organ.

In the case of multiple spots seen on a chest X ray, the causes are even more diverse. The spots would be due to lung cancer only if they result from the original cancer's spread to other parts of the lung. Such spots would indicate that the lung cancer has inevitably spread to other organs also.

WHO IS AT RISK?

Smoking

So uncommon was lung cancer early in this century that some studies seemed to indicate that it had a genetic cause. However, we now know that lung cancer, unlike some other cancers, does not run in families. In cases where several family members had the disease, it is likely they were employed as miners or were exposed to the same occupational risk factors.

In 1939, Drs. Alton Oschner and Michael De Bakey reviewed the first eighty-six patients to undergo surgical removal of a lung cancer. They concluded that "the increased smoking with the custom of inhaling is probably the responsible factor" for lung cancer. In 1967, the United States surgeon general issued the historic report entitled "Smoking and Health." The report summarized the findings of a gathering of the world's leading scientists, the first such assembly devoted entirely to smoking and its harmful effects. Participants included more than 400 scientists from thirty-four countries. Smoking was then, and continues to be, the leading cause of premature death in many countries, resulting not only from cancer but from chronic lung and heart disease. The surgeon general's figures indicate that approximately one-seventh to one-fifth of all Americans now alive—about 28 million people—will die prematurely of diseases caused by cigarettes.

Cigarettes would have been banned years ago were it not for the tremendous economic power of the tobacco lobby. The current attitude of the American government toward cigarettes reflects the $6 billion in annual tax revenues, the political influence of the southern congressional network, and the curious apathy of the American public. The overseas advertising and promotion of American cigarettes has been subsidized. The United States Department of Agriculture also subsidizes the tobacco industry and sponsors research to improve crop yields, while educational and research activities of the National Cancer Institute receive much less funding. Congress has banned cigarette advertising from broadcasting, but not from print. Sensitive perhaps to the $400 million in advertising revenues generated by the tobacco industry, the press has been hesitant in its duty to give appropriate coverage on the harmful effects of tobacco in general and of cigarettes in particular.

While it is difficult to calculate with precision the financial drawbacks of smoking, it does seem clear that the costs far exceed the tax revenues annually generated by tobacco. These are the income loss and treatment expenses of approximately 100,000 tobacco-associated terminal lung cancer patients and of approximately 200,000 victims of respiratory and cardiovascular diseases caused by smoking. In fact, the income loss of those partially or totally disabled from tobacco-related diseases has been calculated at $19 billion. These economic facts are significant for the individuals who imagine that the loss of tobacco export and internal tax revenue would be harmful to the economy.

In the 1970s, the number of adult men who smoked decreased from 43 percent to 37 percent of the population. However, the number of female smokers decreased only slightly, from 31 to 30 percent. And now that women's smoking habits more closely approximate those of men, the incidence of lung cancer in women—and its cost in human and financial terms—has risen rapidly. Of special concern is smoking among teenagers, which greatly increased in the 1960s and early seventies.

Luckily, the cancer-causing chemicals found in cigarette smoke are relatively weak and usually require more than ten years of exposure to bring about a malignant change. Eighty-five percent of lung cancer patients have been smoking for twenty years or more before the diagnosis of cancer.

The Low-Tar, Low-Nicotine Myth

Though the association between cigarette smoking and lung cancer is undeniable, it is still unclear exactly which components of tobacco smoke produce lung cancer. Cigarette smoke is a complex mixture of several thousand different compounds, many of which have been shown either to cause cancer or to promote other cancer-causing agents.

Experimentation with animals is not definitive in studying the effects of these chemicals, since, even when trained for this purpose, the animals do not smoke quite like humans, particularly when it comes to inhaling deeply. In general, tar is responsible for taste, while nicotine is more responsible for the physiologic effect, such as the increased heart rate. To make another generalization: tars are carcinogenic, while nicotine is more responsible for the atherosclerosis, or hardening of the arteries, that leads to greater numbers of heart attacks and strokes.

With the percentage of Americans who smoke decreasing annually, the tobacco industry continues to advertise low-tar cigarettes to keep Americans using a product that is supposedly safer than the high-tar and high-nicotine brands. For example, $150 million has been spent in the campaign to advertise the low-tar, low-nicotine Barclay cigarettes, produced by the Brown and Williamson Tobacco Company.

An article appearing in the *New England Journal of Medicine* in 1983 showed that low-tar, low-nicotine tobacco actually produced significantly higher levels of tar and nicotine than advertised. The low-tar, low-nicotine numbers were derived from tests conducted on smoking machines. Needless to say, machines smoke no more like humans than do animals. The article pointed out that Barclay, Kool Ultra, and Kool Ultra 100's—popular low-tar cigarettes—have filters that contain four channels to lead air directly into the smoker's mouth, where it is supposed to mix with and dilute the smoke during inhalation. In the smoking machine, the air coming through the channels mixing with smoke from the cigarette yielded only 1 mg of tar. However, it has been found that the pressure of the smoker's lips is enough to partially or completely collapse these ventilation channels, thereby impeding the flow of outside air. The real tar delivery appears to be three to seven times higher than that advertised. Barclay may be a success because it does not taste "low-tar."

Another 1983 review, this one by the National Academy of Sciences, showed that smokers of low-tar, low-nicotine brands tended to smoke more cigarettes and to increase the depth and frequency of puffing in an apparent effort to offset the reduction of nicotine and tar. Thus the supposed benefit of switching from a standard cigarette to one of lower tar and nicotine is negated by the smokers' habits.

Smokers of low-nicotine cigarettes do not have a lower risk of heart attack than smokers of cigarettes with higher nicotine levels, and there is no reason to think that the introduction of such cigarettes will decrease the cancer incidence. There has been no drop in lung cancer death rates in *any* country since the introduction of filtered cigarettes or, more recently, of low-tar, low-nicotine cigarettes.

Second-hand Smoke

If a parent, brother, sister, or child has cigarette-induced lung cancer, the risk for the related nonsmoker is three times greater than the risk for the average nonsmoker. Researchers believe this is caused by the carcinogenic effects of smoke in the household atmosphere. In 1981, two significant studies found greater lung cancer risks in the nonsmoking wives of smoking husbands than in the non-smoking wives of nonsmoking husbands. The permanent damaging effects, to say nothing of the cost to society, of such passive or secondhand smoke has barely been recognized.

Asbestos

Lung cancer is extremely common among people who have worked with asbestos, many of whom smoke. For unknown reasons, cigarette smoke combined with asbestos provides a multiplied, rather than additive, risk. The average smoker, in comparison to the general population, runs a ten- to twenty-five-fold increased risk of lung cancer; the average nonsmoking asbestos worker runs only a fivefold increase. The smoking asbestos worker, however, has been found to run a fifty-three-fold increase. Those asbestos workers who smoke heavily—two or more packs per day—run an eighty-seven-fold increase. Unfortunately, more than half of all blue collar workers—and thus, more than half of all asbestos workers—smoke.

Asbestos is a mineral that occurs naturally as a kind of soft rock composed of compressed fibers, and its composition varies in regard to the amount of magnesium, iron, and silicate it contains. One of the best insulators known, it protects from heat, corrosion, and electrical damage. Asbestos fibers can be spun, made into felt, or bonded with other substances. It has been widely used in insulating buildings, boilers, pipes, automobile brake linings and clutch plates, and has even been incorporated into cement as a strengthening agent. Asbestos filters have been used in the manufacture of some imported wines. For many years, hair dryers were insulated with this material. Until recently, asbestos was incorporated into the spackling and taping compounds used for dry wall construction, especially in schools and public buildings. From 1946 to 1973, asbestos was added to spray-on wall coatings used in lieu of plaster. An estimated 30 million tons of asbestos has been used in the United States.

Asbestos produces disease for the most part only when inhaled. It appears to create problems solely because of its tiny size and particular shape. The tiny fibers cannot be easily broken down for removal. Were the fragments larger, they would drop from the airflow in the larger airways that are better equipped to remove such substances, instead of loading in the smaller airways. The typical needle-like shape of asbestos crystals, for unknown reasons, also seems a significant cause of damage. Unfortunately, many of the possible substitutes for asbestos, such as the newer types of fiberglass, may also cause disease if the fibers are of similar size and shape.

A few decades after asbestos dust is inhaled, it can cause three types of diseases: lung cancer, asbestosis, and mesothelioma. Lung cancer is the most common cause of death among those exposed to asbestos. Asbestosis, which occurs *only* in people who have actually worked with asbestos, is a kind of scarring process within the lung itself and on its outer surface. The most common disease produced by exposure to asbestos, it causes the air spaces to become smaller and the lung itself more rigid. Breathing is difficult, waste gases are poorly exchanged, and lung infections are frequent. Mesothelioma, the third disease, is a highly malignant tumor that arises from the lining of the chest wall. Up to forty years or more can elapse between exposure to, and the appearance of, mesothelioma.

Asbestos manufacturing and processing companies now face lawsuits filed by workers suffering from asbestos-related diseases. Ironically, even though cigarettes kill a million smokers (from cancer and cardiovascular disease) every three years, the tobacco industry has never been held liable for a single death.

Other Industrial Agents

Exposure to arsenic also appears to increase lung cancer risk. Arsenic is used more widely than one might think—in the manufacture of glass, pigments, pesticides, and paint—and approximately 1.5 million workers receive occupational exposure. Occupations involving exposure to chromium, solvents from coal or petroleum products, and radiation from uranium mining, may also increase the risk of lung cancer.

Studies conducted by the National Cancer Institute show higher lung cancer rates in northern cities and along the Gulf Coast from Texas to Florida. In general, farming areas have lower rates than industrial areas. Counties with the specific industries of paper, chemicals, petroleum, and shipbuilding have somewhat higher lung cancer rates than counties with other industries, and smokers who work in these industries may be at even higher risk.

Patients Cured of Lung Cancer

Patients fortunate enough to be cured of lung cancer are at high risk for developing a second and separate lung cancer, because the remaining lung has also been subjected to cancer-causing agents. Considering that, statistically, the risk from cigarette smoking is 10 percent, those smokers cured of one lung cancer are estimated to have at least that much risk of developing a subsequent lung cancer. In fact, the incidence of a second lung cancer is even higher, depending on the kind of the original cancer, whether the patient has stopped smoking, and other factors.

Preventive Measures

For most people, prevention of lung cancer is straightforward: don't smoke. For anyone able to stop smoking, every passing year, month, or even day reduces the risk of lung cancer. Damaged and abnormal cells are gradually repaired and replaced over the years. After about ten years of not smoking, the ex-smoker reduces the risk to that of a person who has never smoked! No one can use the excuse that she has been smoking too much and too long for the effort to be worthwhile. Stopping will *always* lower the risk.

Addiction to nicotine can now be satisfied by nicotine chewing gum, available by prescription. The amount per stick is roughly equivalent to that of one cigarette. The substance is quickly absorbed through the lining of the mouth, producing the same "rush" as experienced with the deep inhalation of cigarette smoke. And while nicotine ingested by chewing gum rather than by smoking may cause cardiovascular disease, it will not cause chronic respiratory ailments, such as emphysema or lung cancer.

In a cancer-suspect industry, the industrial environment must be measured by frequent air samplings. Workers should ask to have these measurements posted. If a woman in such an industry cannot stop smoking, ideally she should forsake that employment. Given the compounding of risks of smoking and exposure to possible carcinogens, a woman who has smoked within the past several years and does work involving such industrial exposure is at a significant risk.

Vitamin A is known to mature or differentiate all types of lining, or epithelial, cells toward their specialized, given function. Decreased differentiation, which may be the result of a vitamin A deficiency, is considered a step along the way to malignancy. Five out of six studies showed that individuals with diets or blood levels low in vitamin A have an increased risk of developing lung cancer.

It is possible, however, that higher vitamin A intake is simply an indication of overall better self-care, and that factors other than a vitamin A deficiency are responsible for the increased incidence. Moreover, in several areas of the world—India, the Middle East, Africa—there is no general increase in cancer, or specific increase in lung cancer, despite diets deficient in vitamin A.

The recommended daily allowance of vitamin A is 5,000 I.U. (international units). Being a fat-soluble vitamin, it is not easily discharged from the body, and an excess may cause damage to the liver, bones, and eyes. Since as little as 50,000 I.U. has caused poisonous side effects in some individuals, people taking large doses of vitamin A should have frequent chemical analyses of the blood for prompt detection of side effects. To be safe, one should never take large doses of vitamin A or its precursor, β-carotene (beta-carotene). On the other hand, one can safely increase consumption of foods naturally high in A: yellow vegetables (carrots, sweet potatoes, pumpkins, squash), dark green leafy vegetables (spinach, swiss chard), yellow and orange fruits, liver, and butter. Cabbage, broccoli, cauliflower, and brussels sprouts contain high levels of β-carotene.

DETECTION AND DIAGNOSIS

Chest X Ray

While a simple stethoscope can reveal much about the lungs, it is not especially helpful in diagnosing lung cancer. In this area, the chest X ray is the cornerstone of diagnostic evaluation. The X-ray beam is much like a light beam, except that the invisible energy is far more intense and registers different X-ray densities, depending on the body part through which it passes. The film image shows the bone as white, shows air-filled organs (e.g., the lungs) as black, and all other structures as shades of gray. A cancerous growth, being a solid lump of cells, would exclude air and appear as a gray spot or shadow on the X ray. If the cancer measures less than half an inch, it is difficult to see. Beyond the lungs, the chest X ray supplies information about other chest organs and structures.

A chest X ray normally consists of two views: one from the back to the front, the other from side to side. Both views are necessary to localize any abnormality in three dimensions. The chest X ray itself takes less than a minute. Clothing and especially metal objects, such as necklaces or bras with their fasteners, must be removed to prevent their showing up on the film and obscuring visualization.

Even though the X-ray beam is aimed much higher, the random scattering of X rays to the pelvis may be harmful to an unborn child. In general, the earlier in pregnancy, the greater the potential for harm. Therefore, the abdomen and pelvis should always be protected when a woman is pregnant. In fact, a lead shield might well be used to protect the pelvic area of any woman of childbearing age.

Tomography

Tomography, or laminography, is a technique of X-ray examination by which a number of films are taken, each showing a fraction of an inch slice of lung. All other tissue planes, except the one studied, are blurred and invisible. This exam is useful in determining the presence of additional smaller spots not visible on a simple chest X ray. As mentioned, a finding of multiple spots is unlikely to be caused by lung cancer, and is certainly not early lung cancer.

Mucus, or Sputum, Exam

As the mucus, or sputum, produced deep in the lungs can be cultured to determine whether bacterial or tubercular infection exists, it can also be studied under the microscope to identify cells shed by a cancer. Malignant cells often fall off the tumor bulk at any point in the cancer's growth. The test is positive if malignant cells are found. If normal cells alone are found, either no cancer exists or the tumor had not shed any cells at the time of the sample.

This method of finding early lung cancers is over 80 percent successful in certain research centers. However, some cancers may be situated in small, distant airways where the tumors cannot shed cells to be coughed up in the mucus. Also, only cancer centers doing many such tests are expert enough to find malignant cells this way, especially when they exist only in small numbers. Still, this test is exceptionally valuable in revealing cancerous cells even before the cancer itself can be seen on a chest X ray. The test is painless; the only difficulty a patient may encounter is that of producing a deep lung specimen of mucus and not saliva. Sometimes a patient must inhale a certain mist to loosen a deep mucus sample. Theoretically, any high-risk person is a candidate for this test. Practically, however, the sputum exam is not well enough developed, especially outside of major research centers, to make it effective.

Bronchoscopy

The direct examination of the airway through a slender tube inserted through the nose or mouth is called bronchoscopy. The flexible scope, which can be directed to look into most airways, is so quick and painless that it is usually performed with the patient under local anesthesia. The patient's symptoms or a suspicious chest X ray or sputum exam will often prompt a bronchoscopy as the next test. Unless the patient is short of breath prior to the bronchoscopy, she will have no problem in adequately breathing "around" the bronchoscope. A numbing medicine quiets the cough reflex. There are virtually no complications of bronchoscopy.

Through the bronchoscope, with its special attachments, tissue samples can be taken of any suspicious area. The entire procedure takes about thirty minutes. In addition to biopsies in the airway, a needle may be inserted to pierce and sample lymph nodes or other tissues just beyond the airway. Though complications include bleeding and leakage of air, the procedure in some cases is safer and certainly quicker than an exploratory operation for obtaining the same information.

Bronchography—the inserting of X-ray dye into the airways—is very rarely used to evaluate lung cancer.

CT Scan

Computerized tomography (CT scan) of the chest is highly successful in defining a lung cancer and the extent of its spread into various other structures or organs. This slice-by-slice X ray produces a marvelously accurate cross-sectional image. The test is somewhat uncomfortable, as the patient must lie motionless on a hard table for forty-five to sixty minutes. In addition, the room is kept quite cold in order to provide a proper environment for the computer. Barium is often drunk to outline the food passageway, and dye may be injected intravenously to outline the blood vessels.

Guided by CT or fluoroscopy—the constant X-ray machine—a specialist may insert a long, thin needle through the chest skin, locally anesthetized, precisely into the suspicious mass and withdraw a small sample of cells. This is especially valuable for cancers that are found in small airways, beyond the reach of the bronchoscope. While a quarter of patients experience some air leak, only 10 percent require insertion of a chest tube—also performed under local anesthesia—to withdraw the air and seal the leak.

Mediastinoscopy and Thoracoscopy

If a patient has lung cancer, mediastinoscopy—the visualization of the mediastinum, that part of the chest between the lungs—can help determine whether or not the patient is potentially curable by surgery. Performed under general anesthesia, the procedure usually includes a biopsy of the lymph nodes of the mediastinum. And if lymph nodes on the side opposite that of the lung cancer do not contain malignant cells, a cure by surgery is possible.

In this procedure, after the patient is given general anesthesia, a one-inch incision is made in the lowest part of the neck, just above the breastbone. A lighted viewing instrument is then inserted into the mediastinum. With this procedure, about 35 percent of lung cancer patients are found to have malignant lymph nodes in the mediastinum. Major complications include the rare possibility of puncturing the large blood vessels, which would necessitate chest surgery for repair. Minor complications include air leaks and some bleeding. The procedure takes about an hour. Patients usually leave the hospital two days afterward.

Thoracoscopy is a similar and relatively new surgical procedure. With the patient under general anesthesia, a one-inch incision is made between two ribs and a slender tube, much like a bronchoscope, is inserted into the lung cavity. This procedure permits examination of the entire surface of one lung and of the lining of the chest wall.

Neck Lymph Node Biopsy

Lymph from the lung also drains to the lymph nodes above the collarbone at the base of the neck. If the lymph nodes there are enlarged, and sometimes even if they are not, the physician may recommend their removal for microscopic examination. The procedure is done through a two- to three-inch incision slightly higher and parallel to the collarbone, under either local or general anesthesia. This can be a crucial test, since malignant neck lymph nodes indicate that the lung cancer has spread past the point where it is curable by surgery.

Early Detection

Unfortunately, many smokers believe that with frequent checkups, including chest X rays and physical exams, lung cancer will be detected early enough to allow cure. This is almost never true, because once the malignancy has started, it may take several years before the cancerous cells have multiplied and produced sufficient numbers to be seen on an X ray. By the time it can be seen, the cancer has often spread to other organs. And once apparent on a chest X ray, the course of the disease is usually explosive, with some 50 percent surviving less than six months and less than 10 percent surviving five years. Furthermore, the recent guidelines of the American Cancer Society (ACS) do not recommend routine chest X rays in persons without symptoms.

In deciding these guidelines, the ACS has undoubtedly taken into consideration the cost-to-benefit ratio. "Cost" means exactly that: the costs ($30 to $50) for an annual chest X ray of high-risk American citizens, including 54 million smokers. The benefits entail the number of people who would profit—and the degree to which they would profit— from such tests as an annual chest X ray.

There is every reason to believe that routine chest X rays might result in an earlier detection and increased cure rate. It has been estimated that many lung cancers are visible on a chest X ray twenty months before they cause symptoms. However, one significant study done between 1951 and 1955 found that the costs are large and the benefits relatively small. In the Philadelphia Pulmonary Neoplasm Research Project, more than 6,000 men had biannual chest X rays. The men who were found to have lung cancer had a five-year survival rate of only 8 percent, which approximates that of the general lung cancer population who did not receive frequent routine chest X rays. There are, however, many valid criticisms of this study, including the fact that some men did not undergo the screening as planned and that others diagnosed with lung cancer refused treatment. Another study, this one with 29,000 participants, compared a group with biannual chest X rays to a group with chest X rays every three years. The lung cancer patients diagnosed in the biannual X-ray group had a five-year survival rate of 15 percent; those diagnosed in the once-in-three-years X-ray group had a five-year survival rate of 6 percent.

Three programs studying the benefits of a routine sputum exam combined with a chest X ray for early detection are currently in progress at the widely respected institutions of Johns Hopkins, the Mayo Clinic, and Memorial Sloan-Kettering. Each program has enrolled about 10,000 smokers. Based on the results from these trials, the American Cancer Society is expected to change its guidelines concerning routine chest X rays and/or sputum cytology.

I have painted a rather bleak picture for smokers who wish to continue smoking and persist in the hope that early detection may suffice. However, it would not be honest, or even possible, to present the facts otherwise.

Staging

Not all of the tests described are necessary to prove that the patient has lung cancer. However, a biopsy is essential. A determination of the kind of lung cancer can be very important in selecting the best treatment. In particular, small cell cancer, which constitutes almost 20 percent of lung cancers, is treated rather specially. Some tests are necessary not for the diagnosis but for the cancer's staging (i.e., determining the extent of the disease at the time of diagnosis).

TREATMENT

Surgery

Surgery is the method of cure for all lung cancers other than small cell. Since lung cancer tends to spread so rapidly, it is important to have thorough testing and staging before having part or all of one lung removed. In addition to the tests listed, blood tests and/or scans will investigate the spread to distant organs. An operation to remove lung cancer is major surgery and is not usually performed unless there is a prospect of cure. If the cancer has already spread to the lymph nodes in the neck, to the opposite lung, or distant organs, the surgery will not be curative.

It is estimated that only 20 to 25 percent of all patients qualify for curative surgery. The others have already spread or are medically unfit for the required surgery. The eventual cure rate of those who undergo surgery is only 25 to 30 percent, even if the cancer can be totally removed and there is no known spread at the time of the operation.

Before the operation, two tests are given to determine whether the patient can breathe adequately with some lung tissue removed. An arterial blood sample is obtained from the wrist, elbow, or groin, where a pulse is felt to guide the blood drawer. The arteries lie deeper than the veins and the process is slightly more painful. (Remember that almost all other blood drawing is from the vein.) The arterial blood comes more directly from the lungs than does venous blood, and so the rate of oxygenation and waste gas exchange can be evaluated.

Pulmonary function testing determines the air-moving ability of the lung. The patient inhales and then exhales as fully as possible into a mouthpiece connected to a computerized machine. The patient next breathes in and out as deeply and as frequently as possible, according to the respiratory technician's instructions. With other, similar, breathing maneuvers, the lung reserve is evaluated. The tests are exceptionally important, since smoking may have damaged lung function to some degree. Sadly, some patients have curable cancers but are still unable to undergo lung removal because of poor lung capacity.

If it appears that chest surgery may be curative, the surgeon will try to remove the cancer-containing lobe of the lung with its draining lymph nodes. If the cancer is closer to the central airway, the whole lung may require removal. With the patient lying on the operating table on the unaffected side, a more or less horizontal incision is made between the ribs of the affected side, just under the shoulder blade. The length of time for the procedure varies, with four hours the average. Patients usually remain in the hospital for ten to fourteen days.

Needless to say, there are the usual risks of complications from an extensive surgical procedure.

Radiation

X-ray treatments can be given to patients whose general condition, or more often, whose lung function, prohibits surgery. The X-ray treatment must be directed toward the smallest lung volume possible, while still encompassing the cancer, since X-ray induced scarring and further loss of lung function are likely. Such symptoms as pain, trouble swallowing, and coughing up blood will be relieved in 50 to 80 percent of patients just by shrinking the tumor. A small percentage of people treated by X ray survive five years and are considered cured.

Occasionally, X-ray treatments are given to shrink a cancer before it is surgically removed. X-ray treatment is also often given postoperatively, especially if the cancer has spread to any lymph nodes, in an attempt to improve the cure rate. In addition, if at the time of surgery, the cancer cannot be removed, the physician may implant it with short-distance, high-dose radioactive seeds. This should allow a higher dose of X ray to the cancer while sparing the surrounding lung. This procedure is performed only at major cancer centers, where it is being carefully evaluated.

Chemotherapy

Except in small cell cancer, chemotherapy for lung cancer has been only marginally successful. However, new drugs are always being investigated and more effective drugs will, it is hoped, be found. The primary drugs used are doxorubicin hydrochloride (Adriamycin), cyclophosphamide (Cytoxan), or methotrexate (Folex or Mexate), all of which were developed for use in the treatment of other cancers.

SMALL, OR OAT, CELL CANCER

Small, or oat, cell cancer is unique in that virtually no patients have disease limited to the lung; if the diagnosis of small cell cancer is made, surgery is not attempted. Luckily, this type of cancer is much more sensitive to X ray and chemotherapy than the others, with some long-term survivals and cures. The pretreatment staging tests of small cell cancer are more extensive because of its known tendency to spread rapidly. Evaluation of bone, brain, and liver are routinely performed. Even the bone marrow is sampled, since a quarter of all small cell lung cancer patients have such spread at time of diagnosis.

Given the effectiveness of chemotherapy in this disease, about 10 to 25 percent of patients with limited small cell cancers have prolonged survivals amounting to possible cure. The intensive chemotherapy is administered in a fashion similar to the treatment of acute leukemia, where aggressive drug treatment in conjunction with sophisticated supportive care are commonplace. The actual regimens involve concentrated combinations of three or more drugs, each of which is chosen to kill cancer cells in a different way. Doxorubicin hydrochloride (Adriamycin), cyclophosphamide (Cytoxan), vincristine sulfate (Oncovin), CCNU or Lomustine CeeNU, and/or methotrexate (Folex or Mexate) are frequently used. The drug regimen should be administered by a physician thoroughly trained in the technique.

Cancers of the Skin

Skin cancers are divided into the "common" skin cancers, which arise from basal and squamous (scaly) cells, and the rarer and more dangerous melanoma, which arises from the cells that produce melanin, the substance that gives coloring to the skin.

Basal and Squamous Cell Cancers

Basal and squamous skin cancers—the "common" skin cancers—are the most frequently occurring cancers in the United States, comprising more than an estimated 300,000 cases each year. Since these cancers are most often easily treated in a single visit to a doctor's office, and since cancer rates are based on hospital reporting, the actual incidence may be much higher than estimated. One researcher has calculated that half of all people who live to seventy years of age will experience a skin cancer. Basal and squamous cell cancers spread so infrequently to other areas—in contrast to a rare skin cancer called melanoma—that some may question their malignancy. Nevertheless, if not treated, their continuous growth invades and destroys the surrounding normal tissue.

111

Although they arise from different cells, basal and squamous skin cancers are as similar in treatment as they are in appearance. Squamous cancer originates in flat-shaped cells at the surface of the skin. These cells normally produce keratin, a protein contributing to the protective barrier of the skin.

SYMPTOMS OF COMMON SKIN CANCER*

- A flat, scaly, reddish, or white patch.
- An elevated nodule, usually waxy or pink.
- A hard, flat patch.
- Bleeding or scabbing.

SYMPTOMS

Squamous cell cancer usually appears as a flattish red patch with visible scales or white crusts on the surface. It may also appear as a firm, red nodule with scales. In the faster growing variety, scaling is occasionally absent.

Basal cell cancer originates from round-shaped cells normally located deeper in the skin. This cancer is typically a circular, waxy, dome-shaped nodule, looking somewhat like a wart. It is often translucent, with an overall color often similar to that of the surrounding skin. One can often detect tiny capillaries near the surface. Occasionally, there are various amounts of pigment in the form of small black dots. As the cancer grows, the center becomes depressed and produces an open sore usually covered with a scab. Basal cell cancers can sometimes take other forms, such as a hard, nonelevated skin patch.

Both basal and squamous cancers are, for the most part, not painful. Squamous cancer appears most frequently on the highly sun-exposed areas, such as the back of the hands and the highest parts of the forehead, ears, and nose. However, it can also arise at the skin line of the lower lip or in scars from burns or X-ray treatments from previous decades. (In these areas the squamous cancer will still appear as described.) The disease is more aggressive in such lip/scar sites and may, at times, spread to the draining lymph nodes.

The more common form of basal cell cancer—the waxy nodule with or without ulceration—is found most often on the head and neck, and only 10 percent of the time on the trunk. The less common basal cell cancer form appears frequently on the skin of the chest, upper back, or trunk in general. Basal cell cancers of any type virtually never spread

---

*Look for these especially on face, ears, shoulders, backs of hands, and all sun-exposed areas. Also, look carefully at areas of burn scars or previous X-ray treatment.

to other sites. However, they are capable of invading thoroughly, through the fat, bone, and into the brain, causing death in the few patients who have ignored the continued visible growth over a period of years.

There are no visible premalignant conditions that precede basal cell cancer, although the tumor is usually seen in areas with skin damage from ultraviolet light (i.e., sun) or X rays. In the case of squamous cell, as with many other cancers, there can be a premalignant *in situ* stage. The *in situ* cells look as abnormal microscopically as any actual cancer, but they have not invaded normal tissue—skin, in this case. An *in situ* cancer often appears identical to an actual cancer.

Actinic ("solar") keratoses ("making keratin," as do squamous cells) are rough, reddish, slightly scaly patches only barely raised from the skin's surface and are always found in sun-exposed skin. Some researchers believe that most squamous cancers occurring on sun-exposed skin arise in areas of actinic keratoses. However, actinic keratoses are so common among older individuals who have spent much time in the sunlight, that very few of these ever progress to actual cancer. In fact, they are often so numerous in an affected individual as not to be worth attempting removal. In younger patients, chemotherapy cream may be useful. One to 5 percent 5-FU (fluorouracil) cream or lotion, applied for several weeks, currently seems to be an effective method and the one generally producing little or no permanent scarring.

WHO IS AT RISK?

Ultraviolet light from the sun is the greatest contributing factor in basal and squamous skin cancers. Because sunlight has also been blamed in the case of melanomas, this factor will be discussed later. The people most likely to develop skin cancers are those most prone to sun damage—that is, those with the lightest skin. Prevention involves either complete avoidance of sunlight or protection with sunscreens and sun blocks. Since appearance of one cancer usually signifies sun-exposed skin, other skin cancers are likely to appear on the same individual for the same reason. X-ray treatments for any reason will predispose the treated area to squamous skin cancers. Although rare in any event, this consequence was more likely with the older X-ray machines of two and three decades ago.

DIAGNOSIS AND TREATMENT

Most skin cancers are found and treated when they are one-quarter to one-half inch in size. Even if somewhat larger, the most cosmetic, convenient, and effective treatment is the surgical removal with a tiny margin of normal surrounding skin to ensure removal of the "roots." Biopsy for diagnosis and treatment are thus accomplished in one procedure. The scar is made parallel to the naturally occurring wrinkle lines, or is even placed within a wrinkle, all but concealing it.

If the cancer is larger than half an inch and a skin graft or flap would be needed to close the incision, a small section, encompassing only part of the skin abnormality, is often taken first. In this way, the physician will know exactly what kind of cancer is involved—providing the part removed is representative of the whole—and can better plan the extent of treatment.

Depending upon the area involved, surgery may not produce the best result; for example, on the eyelids, *radiation therapy* is chosen in the majority of cases. The eye itself must be protected from X rays by a small, specially designed lead shield because the lens may otherwise develop a cataract. *Curettage* is a treatment used only for basal cell cancers, which are more amenable to cure than are squamous. After a local anesthesia is administered to the area, a tiny, sharp-edge spoon, or curette, is used to scoop out the cancer. The basal cancer is softer and lacks cohesiveness, whereas the normal tissue is firmer. The base of the scooped and scraped area may be treated with electrocoagulation, and then the charred, coagulated tissue is again scraped out. The depression heals by itself over several weeks. The serious disadvantage of this type of treatment is that no tissue margins are available for microscopic confirmation as to complete removal. *Cryosurgery,* or freezing, also has the same disadvantage. With this technique either liquid nitrogen is sprayed at the cancer or a hollow needle through which liquid nitrogen circulates is inserted into the tumor. The frozen tissue thaws and swells somewhat, followed in a day by the formation of a blister. The dead tumor gradually sloughs away, leaving an open sore in a depressed area. Healing from the edges, which begins to occur within a week, is usually complete by three to four weeks for lesions on the face, but takes longer in other areas, such as the back. *Moh's chemosurgery* involves painting strong chemicals directly on the cancer, followed by horizontal shaving of the area and immediate testing by frozen section. This procedure is used mainly in special instances on cancers of unusual extent and poorly defined margins or on recurrences after previous therapies. There are very few dermatologists in the United States qualified in Moh's chemosurgery. Depending on the size of the cancer, this procedure may take two or more sessions. The depressed open sore that is left at the end of the treatment heals by itself over several weeks.

Although basal cell cancer virtually never spreads to other sites, squamous cell cancer does spread in a small percentage of cases—usually to the nearby lymph nodes. This kind of spread usually occurs only with large and long-ignored cancers. If the lymph node area draining the cancer site is enlarged, removal of that lymph node area is recommended. After the lymph nodes, the most likely site of spread is the lungs.

While the cure rate of these cancers exceeds 95 percent, and the death rate is less than 1 percent, the time, effort, expense, and cosmetic concerns of treatment are considerable.

Melanoma

Melanoma may be considered the opposite of basal and squamous skin cancers. While the latter two appear as skin-colored lumps or open sores, melanoma first appears as a dark spot. In the United States, annual incidence of melanomas is 14,000 cases—1 percent of all cancers—with men and women having the same incidence; the other two skin cancers combined account for more than 300,000 cases each year. While basal and squamous skin cancers rarely spread and cause virtually no deaths, melanomas, because they may spread to other organs, are fatal to about half the people in whom they are diagnosed. These differences are outlined in Table 2.

Melanoma, like all other cancers, is thought to originate from a single cell that becomes malignant and rapidly reproduces itself. In melanoma, that cell is the melanocyte, which produces melanin, the dark pigment that accounts for all skin color. The amount of melanin determines differences in skin tone. Even a woman with light skin and blond hair has melanin; if she did not, her skin would be even lighter, as with albinos. Melanin acts as a protective barrier by absorbing and scattering the sun's ultraviolet rays. A suntan is merely the result of an extra production of melanin through stimulation by the sun.

A mole, or nevus (plural: nevi), is the term used to describe a visible concentration of melanin. There are two kinds of moles: con-

Table 2. Skin Cancers

Melanoma	*Basal and Squamous*
Dark spot	Skin-colored lump or sore
Rare	Common
Sunlight probable factor	Sunlight definite factor
Distributed over the body	Location is 90 percent on the face

genital and acquired. As the name indicates, congenital moles are present at birth; acquired moles appear later, usually in adolescence or later. Few babies are born with more than one mole, but by adulthood the average white person has twenty-five to forty acquired moles. The average black person has none at birth and acquires very few with age. Although melanomas may be found anywhere on the body, the most frequent sites are the upper back and shoulders in both sexes and the calves in women. Roughly a third of all melanomas occur on the legs, another third on the head and neck area, and another third on the arms and trunk.

SYMPTOMS OF MELANOMA

- Any skin spot that changes in any way (growth, bleeding, itching, etc.).
- Any dark spot with irregular margins, varying elevations, or more than one color.

SYMPTOMS

While most people are aware that any mole that bleeds and/or forms scabs should be removed, it is important to realize that *any* change—in the size, color, elevation, or sensitivity—of a mole is suspicious. By the time a mole has begun to bleed, melanoma cells have already invaded deeply enough to reach the skin's blood vessels. Therefore, any alteration in any characteristic of a mole should be brought to a doctor's attention. Sometimes, however, especially in the dormant stage of early melanomas, changes occur so slowly that they are virtually undetectable.

Nonetheless, there are ways of finding suspicious moles. Even if a woman has not noticed a specific change in a given mole, she can examine its present coloration, border, and surface. Most benign moles have a uniform color throughout, but an early melanoma may have more than one color, including navy blue, reddish brown, brown, and black. Navy blue is the color that should arouse greatest suspicion. Most benign moles have a regular circular periphery; one that should cause concern might have an irregular, notched border and resemble spilled coffee or an ink stain. Finally, while most benign moles have a smooth surface, an early melanoma may exhibit slightly different elevations. Often, these changes can be felt as a bumpy surface more readily than they can be seen, although varying elevations can be detected best by observing the mole's surface in profile.

Thus, in addition to actual changes, each mole should also be evaluated for variegated color, border irregularity, and surface differ-

Table 3. Melanoma Self-Exam

Finding	Action	
	Repeat Exam in Six Months	See Doctor
Appearance of "new" mole		X
"Old" moles:		
No change	X	
Any change		X
Circular	X	
Irregular border		X
Smooth surface	X	
Varying surface		X
Single color	X	
More than one color		X

ences. These characteristics are apparent in the following photographic enlargements of early melanoma.

Somewhat less than one-half of all melanomas start in preexisting moles. The remainder arise from newly pigmented spots on apparently normal skin. These spots strongly resemble an ordinary mole. Therefore, in addition to observing one's known moles, one should also take note if any new moles arise. Any true mole that arises after early adulthood, around age twenty or later, should be removed. However, "aging spots," which look like small, light brown freckles, are not true moles and are not usually suspicious.

If one has many moles, it is difficult to remember their exact positions and sizes in order to note new moles or the growth of old ones. For greatest certainty, it is best not to trust your memory, but to construct a chart or map of the skin. This is how I and other doctors record moles on patients for the sake of comparison from year to year. In addition to the steps listed on the mole map, one can trace the larger moles with transparent paper instead of measuring them.

Almost all melanomas originate on the skin's surface, but 2 to 5 percent of this rare disease begins elsewhere (e.g., in the eye, the salivary glands, the lining of the inside of the mouth). Most of the time, even in these unusual locations, a melanoma will first appear as a black spot. The areas under the fingernails and toenails are also possible sites, and melanomas are often mistaken for a bruise, such as with a smashed fingertip.

Research indicates that rare, dime-sized or larger (1.5 cm) congenital moles are most likely to become melanomas. Research also indicates that smaller congenital moles are more likely to become

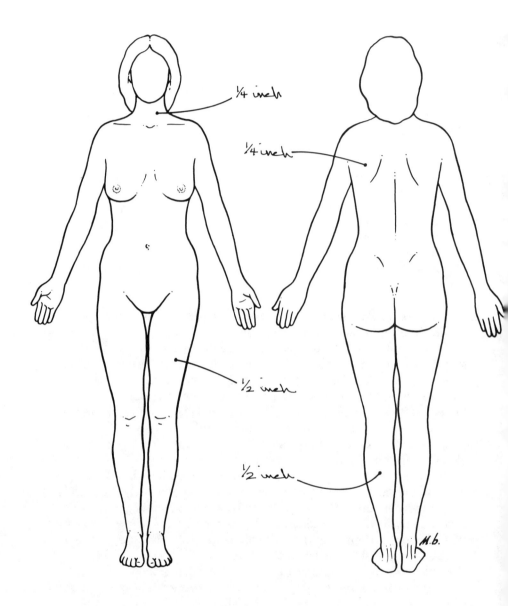

MOLE MAP
1. *Draw two complete body outlines—front and back.*
2. *Measure your moles with a ruler, and draw the mole in its position with the size measurement next to it.*
3. *Keep the map to check if a mole is new or if an old one has grown.*

melanomas than adulthood, or acquired, moles—though this is not as certain. Most studies confirm that 10 percent of large congenital moles prove malignant, though some have found the rate to be as high as 30 percent.

How can you tell if you were born with a large mole or if it appeared in later life—that is, whether it is congenital or acquired? Any mole larger than 1.5 cm (the size of a dime) is almost always congenital. Acquired moles are simply not that big. On the other hand, even experienced doctors cannot usually judge from appearance which are small congenital moles and which are acquired moles.

Along with most doctors who see many patients with melanomas, I recommend removal of all congenital moles. Obviously, if removal is likely to result in a disfiguring scar, one might wish to accept the risk of a future malignancy by not having it removed. However, if a congenital mole is not removed, it should be examined periodically for variegated color, irregular border, and surface differences. And, if danger signs appear, the mole should be removed at once.

As long as the mole is uniform throughout, and the biopsied part is typical of the remainder—though no doctor can really guarantee that—biopsy of only part of the mole should suffice to determine malignancy. If the mole is suspicious enough to be biopsied, however, any doctor would prefer to remove it all to prevent future malignant change.

WHO IS AT RISK?

While some cancers, such as breast cancer, do have a tendency to run in families, any genetic predisposition to melanoma is slight. Only 6 to 10 percent of all melanoma patients report a blood relative with the disease.

Although the cause/effect relationship between sunlight and melanoma is weaker than that between it and common skin cancers, sunlight is still the only known important cause of melanomas. The strength of ultraviolet rays, the damaging component of sunlight, varies with closeness to the equator, altitude, and, of course, the time of day and season. All other factors—hours spent in sunshine, for example—being equal, melanoma incidence varies in proportion to one's proximity to the equator. An Australian study illustrated this point. The light-skinned immigrants to that continent experienced an increased incidence of melanoma in direct proportion to the distance that they lived from the equator.

In the United States, the incidence of all skin cancers—including melanomas—increases in proportion to greater amounts of sunlight. In Texas, for example, there were 73 cases of skin cancer per 100,000 population in 1978; in New York, 58 cases per 100,000; and in Alaska, 34 cases per 100,000. For every 3,000 feet above sea level, there is a 15 percent increase in the strength of ultraviolet rays due to the thinning atmospheric "filter." This may be an important factor in a city such as Denver, which is approximately one mile above sea level.

Although still quite rare, melanoma appears to be the cancer with the greatest recent increase. In the past twenty years, the number of cases has almost doubled. Though no one knows exactly why the incidence of melanoma has increased so rapidly, most cancer experts feel that increased ultraviolet ray damage is the most important factor. The most common skin sites for melanomas are those most commonly exposed to the sun: the upper back and shoulders of men and women and the calves of women, which are exposed when women wear skirts. The increased occurrence over the past two decades is not surprising when one considers that swimming pools, vacations on the beach, and ultraviolet ray tanning salons were generally unavailable in the 1940s and 1950s, and that more skin was covered and protected before current bathing suit fashions. Furthermore, not until recently has there been such a desire for the "healthy," tanned appearance, symbolizing the leisure and means to play in the sun.

In addition to the increased hours people spend basking in the sun, sunlight is gradually becoming more powerful. The ozone layer high in the atmosphere partly shields the earth from damaging ultraviolet sunrays. But chlorofluorocarbons, the gaseous contents of aerosol spray cans and refrigerators, invade the upper atmosphere and displace and diminish the ozone levels. The oxides of nitrogen and water vapor in the exhaust of supersonic transport planes has the same effect. Both of these are recent phenomena. For every 1 percent decrease in the thickness of the ozone layer, the incidence of general skin cancers increases 4 to 10 percent. There is every reason to suspect that melanoma, in particular, increases for the same reasons.

Preventive Measures

Because the action of ultraviolet rays is the only known factor in causing melanoma, exposure should be reduced by protecting the skin either with clothing or sun-blocking chemicals such as para-aminobenzoic acid (PABA). The higher the concentration of PABA in a sunblock, the better; drugstore preparations contain up to 15 percent PABA. Because PABA tends to stain clothes and washes off with water, it has been replaced in commercial sun-blocks to some extent by newer chemicals, including padimate-O, cinnamates, benzophenones, and salicylates. It is possible that one or another of these might irritate your skin. If a certain brand of block makes your skin red or itchy, try a sunscreen with different chemicals listed as the ingredients.

The ability of these products to protect the skin is usually expressed as a Sun Protection Factor, or a SPF number. The number is a multiple of the time needed for the sun to produce an effect on the skin. A woman who burns in fifteen minutes at high noon would take thirty minutes to acquire the same sunburn while using an SPF 2 sunscreen. With an SPF 8 sunscreen, she could be exposed for two hours before burning.

Alcoholic solutions of the sunscreen are invisible after soaking into the skin. Creams and lotions are also available, but tend to be greasy. The solution should be applied every morning to the face and other exposed parts of the body after washing and before makeup is applied. Unless removed by swimming or sweating, one heavy application will be enough protection for the day. The solution should be applied thirty to sixty minutes before exposure to the sun in order for it to soak in, and it should be applied even though one is wearing a hat. If one sits under a beach umbrella, 50 percent of ultraviolet rays can be reflected by the sand or water. Accordingly, a sunscreen should be used even on cloudy days, since 80 percent of ultraviolet rays can penetrate cloud cover. And even if one is always in the water, it's a good idea to apply sunscreen since as much as 50 percent of ultraviolet rays travel through the water. Sunscreen should also be reapplied after swimming. To be really safe, one should use sunscreen even when wearing regular clothing at the beach, since wet T-shirts, gauzy beach robes, and other lightweight clothing can let through up to 30 percent of the sun's ultraviolet rays.

Athletes should be aware that more ultraviolet rays are present at the high altitudes required for snow skiing and mountain climbing, and that concrete and snow, as well as water and sand, also reflect ultraviolet rays.

While sun-blocks may prevent burning, a suntan alone results in changes to the skin and stimulation of the melanocyte. To reduce risk of skin cancers, it is probably best to avoid sunburning and even suntanning. Ultraviolet ray damage is cumulative. Many short sun exposures add up, and the total may be as damaging as fewer long exposures.

Several studies have noted a higher rate of melanoma in white collar workers than in outdoor workers, such as farmers and construction workers; other studies have demonstrated a higher incidence in people of higher socioeconomic classes. Both of these situations can still be correlated with exposure to sunshine—vacations at a Caribbean beach—while outdoor workers may well have built up a tan slowly by daily exposure over the years. The outdoor workers would be protected against sunburn even though the skin still showed effects of chronic solar damage. The intense, though intermittent, exposure to ultraviolet rays, such as indoor workers are more likely to experience, may trigger melanoma at an increased rate.

Although melanoma arises in melanocytes, the pigment producing cells, the fact that blacks have more pigment does not increase their risk of melanoma. On the contrary, the lightest skinned person—the person with the fewest melanocytes and thereby the least pigment—has the greatest risk of melanoma. Though one tends to think of blue-eyed blondes as the high-risk group, many women with dark hair and dark eyes have equally light skin, with an equally high risk of melanoma. The most reliable indicator of high-risk skin is the tendency to burn instead of tan.

In the rare instance when a darker-skinned person develops melanoma, it often begins in unusual areas. The sites in darker persons are usually, for unknown reasons, the *non*exposed areas. The most common site in American blacks is the sole of the foot. Other sites in dark-skinned individuals include the inside of the mouth, the palm of the hand, and the eyes.

Ultraviolet ray damage aside, other kinds of injuries to moles do not cause melanoma. For instance, were one occasionally to cut a leg mole while shaving, the worst consequence would be the inconvenience. In such cases, removal of the mole is recommended for practical purposes. The same applies to moles under bra straps or belts.

DIAGNOSIS AND TREATMENT

Any change whatever in the outward configuration of a mole should be brought to a doctor's attention immediately. This is especially so, since the danger of a melanoma results more from its depth than from the extent of spread over the skin surface. In other words, depending on the extent to which melanoma has invaded the underlying tissue, a melanoma of one-eighth-inch diameter may be a more dangerous melanoma than one measuring three inches. The ability of a melanoma to spread to other sites is, in fact, directly related to its depth.

Depth can be measured only by surgical removal of the mole and microscopic determination of the melanoma's skin layer penetration. Levels are graded from I to V, with I the most superficial and slowest spreading, and V the deepest and most aggressive. These levels dictate treatment procedure. Patients with the more active melanomas tend to need more treatment, as well as more careful medical observation for the possibility of future spread.

Surgery

There is no question but that electrodesiccating, electrocoagulation, or burning off, a mole (often done on warts) will produce a neater scar. In some areas, this circular scar will look better than the linear scar produced by surgical removal with a scalpel. Electrodesiccation, however, is not an option in removing a mole, because it yields no tissue to be microscopically examined for the presence of melanoma. Freezing, or cryosurgery, is an unacceptable procedure for the same reason.

The only way to be certain of the presence or absence of melanoma is to remove what appears to be a mole and check it microscopically. It is usually not advisable to remove only part of the growth for diagnosis, since it is possible that the biopsied part will be benign, even though the remaining adjacent part is cancerous. Therefore, a suspicious mole is removed completely with only a small border of normal skin around it—perhaps one-eighth of an inch. If the mole is not a melanoma, the small scar, only slightly bigger than the mole itself, will be the end result. If, however, the apparent mole is a melanoma, then a larger amount of tissue must be removed from the former surgical site to prevent regrowth. Melanoma, like most other cancers, has microscopic extensions in the area that may cause a recurrence near the scar unless enough adjacent tissue is also removed. How much surrounding tissue should be removed is a matter of experience and judgment. The surgeon considers the location and the depth of the melanoma, among other factors. On the face, the cosmetic factor is especially significant.

If the melanoma is located in an area with tight skin (e.g., the calf), then a skin graft may be necessary to cover the area. A skin graft may be taken from the front of the thigh or from a less visible area, such as the buttocks, where the graft scars will not show, even in a bathing suit. If the skin is loose, the edges of the wound are simply pulled together, and a skin graft is not necessary. In addition to the skin, it is often necessary to remove some underlying fat, and in some areas this may result in a depressed scar.

Melanoma treatment depends upon the extent of spread when the patient first consults a cancer surgeon. If the melanoma appears localized to the starting spot, treatment involves surgical removal with the surrounding skin and fat. This procedure, usually performed with the patient under general anesthesia, is often all that is necessary.

Enlargement of the lymph glands, or lymph nodes, in the nearest area (armpit, groin, or neck) usually signals the presence of melanoma. Accordingly, the surgeon removes the fat and lymph nodes of that region. If the nearest lymph nodes do not appear enlarged, the surgeon carefully examines the area over the ensuing months and years. The lymph nodes are surgically removed if and when the enlargement occurs.

Occasionally, and under greatly varying circumstances, it may be in the patient's best interest for the lymph nodes to be removed, even without enlargement. If the melanoma has invaded the deepest skin layers (level IV or V), there is good reason to suspect that melanoma has already invaded the lymph nodes, and it may be advisable to remove them preventively, *before* they enlarge. If a patient is too heavy to feel lymph node enlargement or will perhaps be unavailable for a follow-up exam for several months because of travel, removal of what appear to be normal-sized lymph nodes, at time of melanoma surgery, may be the best course.

Special Treatments

X-ray treatment is not frequently used in the treatment of melanoma, because the disease is not particularly responsive to it. Chemotherapy, routinely used for all kinds of cancers, can be administered into the general bloodstream or into the blood flow of a particular limb. Melanoma is one of the few cancers that is somewhat external to the rest of the body, occurring on the leg or arm (to name two of the more common sites). Accordingly, some special treatments are available only for this form of cancer.

When a melanoma appears on the leg, the artery carrying blood to, and the vein carrying blood from, the leg can be exposed in an operation at the groin. Tubes are positioned in the artery for injection of a high-dose anticancer drug that circulates through the leg and is subsequently removed at the vein. During the several hours of the operation, the leg has a high drug concentration (much higher than the rest of the body could tolerate). Because the artery and vein have, in effect, been isolated in a "closed-circuit" arrangement, the drug does not escape to other parts of the body. For that reason, such chemotherapy side effects as nausea, vomiting, and hair loss can be kept to a minimum. This technique is called isolation perfusion.

Since heat damages all cells—and malignant cells more than normal cells—the contents of this blood exchange are sometimes heated so that the leg temperature rises to about 107°F. Normal cell enzymes can routinely repair such heat damage. The enzymes of cancer cells are directed mainly to cell reproduction, so their repair enzymes are weak. A significant number of malignant cells, therefore, are killed by heat alone because they cannot repair themselves.

In addition, melanoma appears to respond better than other cancers to stimulation of the body's own defenses, or immunotherapy. In one type of immunotherapy treatment, a person's own melanoma cells, which stimulate the lymphocytes to develop antibodies, are injected as vaccine. The melanoma cells are first removed and grown in the laboratory. The cells are then "killed"—lest they continue to reproduce—and are injected back into the body. Since it is difficult to grow cells in a laboratory, a vaccine from other patients' melanomas can be used if they grow more successfully than one's own. In another form of immunotherapy treatment, the immune defenses are stimulated not against melanoma specifically, but in general. For example, the vaccine against tuberculosis—BCG (Bacillus Calmette Guerin)—is known to be a general stimulant of the immune system. Beyond its use in countries with large amounts of tuberculosis, BCG has been used with some success against melanoma.

Cancers of the
Head and Neck

The category of cancer commonly referred to as "head and neck" is limited to the lip, inside of the nose, sinuses, mouth, throat, and larynx, or voice box. These cancers differ in cell of origin, diagnosis, and treatment from other cancers, such as skin and thyroid cancers, that are also located in the head and neck. Head and neck cancers, thus defined, originate on the outer layer or lining—areas in contact with cancer-causing agents, both inhaled and swallowed.

About one in twenty cancers diagnosed in the United States will be a head and neck cancer, accounting for 39,000 estimated cases in 1984. Seventy percent of these will be found in men. However, since most head and neck cancers are related to smoking, the percentage of women affected will undoubtedly grow with the increasing number of long-term women smokers.

The lining of the areas affected by head and neck cancer is squamous (scaly) tissue, probably named because the cells are flattish and resemble scales under the microscope. Although this lining is similar to that of the body's external skin, its appearance is different and the cells do not produce keratin, a protein that helps make the exterior skin impermeable to water. Head and neck cancer is a squamous malignancy about 90 to 95 percent of the time. Also interspersed through much of the head and neck lining are hundreds of tiny salivary glands no larger than one-eighth of an inch in diameter. If this gland is the source of the malignancy, the result is an adenocancer, which occurs 5 to 10 percent of the time. Treatment is the same for both types.

Most of the areas of the head and neck, and particularly those that are cancer-prone, are immediately visible either to the individual with a mirror or by means of special mirrored instruments in the doctor's office. Unfortunately, the ease of examination and diagnosis in most of these areas is not reflected in an encouraging cure rate: Somewhat more than a third of those diagnosed die of head and neck cancer.

The structures affected by head and neck cancer are contained in a relatively small area—no larger than a three-inch cube. However, in that compressed area are small, fine muscles responsible, in varying degrees, for the functions of speaking, swallowing, and breathing. In addition, the areas under discussion are found in the face and in the slightly less visible area of the neck. As one may appreciate, the concern in head and neck cancer is not totally one of cure, as is the case with other cancers. Concern for the basic functions of speaking, eating, and breathing, as well as for facial appearance also enters into planning and delivering treatment.

SYMPTOMS OF HEAD AND NECK CANCER

- In the mouth and throat lining, an abnormality, usually painless, which could be
      an open sore, occasionally bleeding;
      a lump;
      a hard, nonelevated patch; or
      a discolored patch.
- Pain or difficulty with swallowing.
- Pain in the ear.
- Hoarseness.
- Rarely: nasal bleeding.

SYMPTOMS

The most common sign of head and neck cancer is an abnormality of the lining, usually appearing as an open ulcer, or sore. The circular edges of the ulcer may be raised and firm. These sores do not usually hurt. The cancer may also appear as a lump, especially in the case of salivary gland cancer, or merely as a hard, nonelevated area. Bleeding may be a sign of the cancer, though not an early sign. Cancers far back in the rear of the mouth or throat are harder for the individual to see or feel and may not be noticed until there is difficulty or pain in swallowing. Since some nerves from the ear connect with those in the throat, ear pain may also be an indicator. Hoarseness may be a sign of cancer at or near the larynx, or voice box. Frequently, nasal bleeding may be a sign of cancer of the nasal cavity, although malignancy at this site is rare in the United States and Europe. Sometimes a head and neck cancer is not suspected until the appearance of one or more lumps in the neck, indicating spread to the lymph nodes. The most common site of spread is the lymph nodes on the same side of the neck as the original cancer.

Of course, there are many reasons, besides cancer, for sores on the lips or inside the mouth, such as the usual canker sore or other minor infections. In contrast to most cancers, these benign sores are usually painful, which leads to their discovery. But since some cancers may also be painful, the presence or absence of discomfort is not a reliable gauge. Any sore that does not completely heal within ten to fourteen days should be called to the attention of a doctor for possible biopsy. The same advice applies to hoarseness or lumps in the neck: anything that persists more than fourteen days should be examined. Though hoarseness, even if long-standing, is likely to be caused by smoking, allergies, or voice abuse—common among singers, teachers, and others whose professions place strain on the voice—it should be checked by a doctor. As is mentioned in the chapter on lymphoma, there are many nonmalignant reasons for enlargement of the neck lymph nodes. These usually involve infections draining to the lymph nodes— for example, strep throat and tooth infections.

Premalignant conditions—with the same causes as cancers—may also at times be visible. A painless, slightly elevated velvety red patch (erythroplakia) is usually the sign of a highly premalignant area, which may contain actual cancer. Slightly elevated or flat, usually painless, white patches, which appear dryer than the surrounding tissue, are called leukoplakia. While leukoplakia is not always precancerous, this cannot be determined without biopsy.

Preventive Measures

Prevention of head and neck cancers starts with self-examination. First, with a well-lit mirror and flashlight, examine and then feel the lips, gums, and inside of the cheeks. Check for any color change (darker red or lighter pink or white), any elevation or depression of the normal level (a lump or ulcer), and any texture changes (an area "harder" than surrounding tissue). Any area that is scabbed, cracked, bleeding, or numb should cause concern. The most likely site for cancer of the lip area is the vermilion border, on the lower lip, where the face and lip skin meet. No one area of the cheek is any more likely than another to develop cancer except in cases of snuff users and tobacco chewers, where the cheek area that routinely comes into contact with these substances is highly prone. Some researchers feel that areas of chronic denture irritation may have a slightly greater tendency to develop cancer than other areas.

Second, check the floor of the mouth, under the tongue, and the roof of the mouth in the same way. The roof of the mouth is generally an unlikely place for the cancer to develop, though the horseshoe-shaped floor of the mouth is quite cancer-prone. This may be due to cancer-causing agents in the saliva, which tend to collect at that site from gravity.

Last, examine the tongue—the tip, the top, the underneath, and the sides—for the same factors, including color changes, depressions, elevations, and hard areas. With a dry cloth, such as a handkerchief, grasp the tip so that you can pull the tongue first out and then in all directions to view every area. Cancer of the tongue is most likely to develop at the tip or sides. Unfortunately, the throat and beyond can barely be seen by the individual herself; likewise, the nasal cavity and sinuses are difficult to examine.

DIAGNOSIS AND TREATMENT

In head and neck cancers that can be seen, a small sample—a sixteenth of an inch or so—can be removed from the surface after administration of a local anesthetic during the initial doctor's office visit. Once cancer has been diagnosed, few tests are necessary before proceeding with treatment. The tendency for spread to distant organs—such as the liver, brain, lungs, and bones—is much less with the general head and neck cancers than with other cancers. Therefore, while other cancers may require multiple scans of various organs to properly stage the patient, head and neck cancer, at least of the common squamous variety, is often completely staged by a chest X ray, blood tests, and evaluation of the extent of the original cancer and its spread, if any, in the neck. This is not to imply that head and neck cancers are not dangerous. The structures in the head and neck are so important that their involvement with cancer can be fatal. In fact, of all patients who die of this disease, almost half have cancer limited to the head and neck with no distant organ involvement.

Surprising though it may seem, the general divisions of the head and neck area—lip, mouth (oral cavity), throat (pharynx), voice box (larynx), nasal part of the throat (nasopharynx), and sinuses—are quite different in diagnosis and treatment and will be discussed separately. As is generally known, tobacco is the main cause of head and neck cancer, except for a few rare sites, such as the nasopharynx and the sinuses. There is no genetic predisposition except possibly in nasopharynx cancer. Stopping smoking can benefit even those patients who have already had a cancer of the oral cavity or larynx. Of those who were cured of their first cancer but continued to smoke, 40 percent developed a second cancer in the head and neck area within seven years. In contrast, only 6 percent of those who quit smoking developed a second cancer.

The Lip

By virtue of its location, the lip is susceptible to the same cancer-causing factors as the facial skin. Prolonged, intense exposure to sunlight and exposure to tobacco are the major causes of lip cancer. Most studies confirm that 60 to 80 percent of lip cancers occur in elderly, fair-skinned white men who work out-of-doors. Lip cancers are rare in blacks; women account for only 10 percent of lip cancers, presumably because they spend less time outdoors and/or are protected from the sun by lipstick and other cosmetics. Ninety-five percent of lip cancers occur on the lower lip, which is more sun-exposed. Studies show that about 80 percent of lip cancer patients smoked tobacco and many smoked a pipe. A risk beyond that of the chemical carcinogens in tobacco may result from the long-term contact with the heat and pressure of a pipe stem.

Because of its visible location, lip cancers are found easily when only one-quarter to one-half inch in size. Even when the cancer is somewhat bigger, surgical removal is the usual treatment. A minute biopsy—surgical removal of a sixteenth of an inch or so—will reveal the malignancy. Curative surgery usually involves removal of the cancer with a surrounding margin of normal skin, followed by plastic surgical repair of the defect. If lip cancer spreads, as occurs in less than 15 percent of cases, its pattern is slightly different than that of other head and neck cancers. It will manifest itself first in enlarged lymph nodes under the chin and only afterward with enlarged lymph nodes in the neck. While radiation therapy is possible, it is not used nearly as often as surgery.

The Mouth (Oral Cavity) and the Throat (Pharynx)

In the United States, cancer of the mouth and throat accounts for no more than 5 percent of all cancers, while in India and some parts of Southeast Asia, the figure ranges from 40 to 50 percent. The specific cancer-causing agent varies culturally and geographically. For example, in India and Pakistan, numerous street vendors sell *pan,* which is a mixture of spices and the leaves and nut of the tobacco-related betel plant. According to users, the physiologic effects include a curbing of the appetite, a feeling of relaxation, and increased salivation. Both men and women use it almost as commonly as we use chewing gum. Residents of Soviet Central Asia, Afghanistan, and nearby countries also have a high incidence and death rate from oral cancer. They chew *nass,* a combination of betel nut or tobacco, lime, and sesame oil. Unfortunately, the habit of chewing tobacco, or other plants with pharmacologic activity, is more or less a worldwide practice.

The portion of the oral cavity affected by cancer corresponds to the area in which the tobacco is held. (Even if tobacco is not chewed, it still affects the lining of the mouth and throat—though in a decreased concentration—as when it is smoked.) More than 90 percent of all oral and pharyngeal cancers occur in patients over forty-five years of age. The incidence increases suddenly with age and there is a sharp rise in the sixty- to sixty-four-year-old group. Generally, women are diagnosed at an earlier age than men. People in low-income groups have higher incidence rates for oral and pharyngeal cancer compared to those in high-income groups; this generally parallels their incidence of smoking.

Persons with leukoplakia and erythroplakia (premalignant conditions) are at high risk for developing a head and neck cancer. Of all mouth and throat cancer patients, almost half have had leukoplakia. On the other hand, leukoplakia is so common that less than 10 percent of all cases will progress to cancer within several years.

Cancers larger than 2 cm (the size of a nickel) are frequently accompanied by enlarged neck lymph nodes, more so in throat cancer than in mouth cancer. Small early cancers (less than 2 cm) are treated well either by radiation or surgery, depending to some extent on the location. Removing so small a cancer on the front two-thirds of the tongue will usually produce no malfunction of speech or swallowing. If the cancer appears on the back third of the tongue, and especially if positioned toward the middle, radiation therapy is the treatment of choice. Radiation is usually employed for cancers of the tonsil, back of the tongue, and wall of the throat, although, if cancers are small enough, surgery can be successful and more convenient. For larger cancers, both radiation and surgery are necessary.

When cancers of the mouth encroach upon the mandible, or jawbone, surgical treatment is often preferable because X-ray therapy may destroy normal bone. For a large (2 cm) cancer of the mouth, surgery may include removal of the original cancer along with the nearby jawbone and neck lymph nodes. Should this include a large amount of mouth or throat, a skin graft, or skin and muscle flap from another area, such as the chest, may be necessary for replacement. Postoperative X-ray therapy or chemotherapy may be administered three to four weeks later to treat any unremoved microscopic extensions. Occasionally, preoperative chemotherapy or X-ray therapy may be helpful. Despite the extensiveness of an operation for so large a cancer, there is virtually no pain; the area is numb due to the severing of the nerves. The scars are extensive on the neck and inside the mouth, but there is usually only one small visible scar in the middle of the lower lip.

The overall cure rate for mouth cancer (including all sites: roof, floor, tongue, gums, and inside of cheeks) is about 50 percent. The overall cure rate for throat cancer (including tonsil, soft palate, and all the lining above the larynx) is about 15 percent.

The Voice Box (Larynx)

The incidence of cancer of the larynx varies worldwide, but invariably predominates in men by an incidence of about eight to one. Larynx cancers represent 2.3 percent of all cancers in men in the United States, and only 0.4 percent of all cancers in females. The number of laryngeal cancers appears to be proportional to the number of lung cancers, with a ratio of one larynx cancer for every ten lung cancers. Cancer of the larynx is primarily a disease of old age, the average age at the time of diagnosis usually being the sixth and seventh decades.

Tobacco use is the major cause of laryngeal cancer. In 1970, in a study of larynxes of men who died of causes other than laryngeal cancer, abnormal, but not malignant, cells were found in 99 percent of the cigarette smokers; in only 20 percent of nonsmokers were there similar findings. In Utah, the larynx cancer rate is only 60 percent of that found generally in the United States. Seventy percent of the residents of the state profess the Mormon religion, which forbids the use of tobacco and alcohol.

In 1956, fifteen times as many men as women were diagnosed for larynx cancer. In 1976, a similar study showed a change in proportion of five men to every woman, suggesting that the increase in female larynx cancer was proportionate to the increase in the number of women smokers generally. Women have "come a long way," indeed!

The rare benign growth involving the actual vocal cords is called papilloma. It occurs with equal frequency among male and female children and usually disappears spontaneously during puberty. In

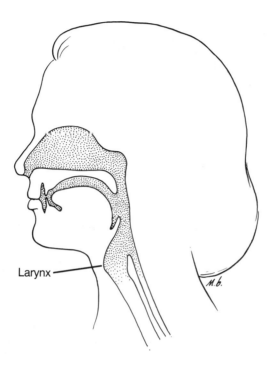

The larynx

adults, it occurs twice as frequently in males as in females. It almost always causes hoarseness and tends to be multiple and recurring after treatment. The papillomas seem to be caused virally and greatly resemble virally caused skin warts. In decades past, laryngeal papillomas were treated with radiation and sometimes became malignant. Radiation is no longer a treatment for this condition. Worldwide, only four cases have been reported of malignancy arising from laryngeal papillomas *not* previously treated by radiation.

Cancers of the larynx are classified into three groups, depending on their site of origin. Those originating slightly above the true vocal cords (supraglottic—"supra" means above and "glottis" means larynx) comprise about 40 percent of laryngeal cancers; those actually on the vocal cords, 60 percent; and those below the true vocal cords, 1 percent. The area above the vocal cords is richly supplied with lymphatic vessels and 60 percent of patients with cancers arising there have enlarged lymph nodes at the time of diagnosis. Hoarseness seldom occurs until late in the course of cancer occurring above the vocal cords; a lump in the neck or ear pain may be the first symptom.

On the other hand, cancer of the true vocal cord itself has the most favorable prognosis, probably because hoarseness is among the earliest symptoms of this curable disease. In addition, the probability of spread to the lymph nodes is small, since the area has few lymphatic vessels. The rare cancer that develops below the true vocal cords does not cause hoarseness, but may cause shortness of breath from partial obstruction of the airway.

In the United States, more than half of all patients with any kind of larynx cancer are diagnosed with the tumor still localized to the larynx. Another 25 percent are not diagnosed until the tumor has progressed to involve the nearby tissues or lymph nodes; another 15 percent, only when the tumor has spread to distant areas.

Early cancers of the larynx can be treated by radiation or surgery. Surgery, consisting of a partial removal of the larynx, usually results in slight but permanent hoarseness. More advanced laryngeal cancers are still quite curable compared to cancers of other sites. Similarly, advanced surgical treatment of later stages of cancer involves removal of the whole larynx (with loss of normal speaking) and the neck lymph nodes, if they are thought to be involved. If a complete laryngectomy is performed, the end of the windpipe, or trachea, is exposed as a hole, or stoma, low in the middle of the neck, via a tracheostomy. Breathing occurs through the new hole instead of through the nose and mouth. More than 75 percent of all patients who require total removal of the larynx develop successful esophageal speech as a replacement for normal laryngeal speech. Air travels through the esophagus (the swallowing tube) instead of through the trachea and larynx, and the words are formed by the mouth and tongue as in normal speech. For the 25 percent whose esophageal speech is partly or totally unsatisfactory, a battery-powered buzzer may be pressed onto the neck. The sound waves formed by the buzzer are transmitted through the mouth and shaped into sounds and words by moving the lips and tongue in the usual way. Although understandable, the result is a flat-sounding, electronics-generated voice.

Compared to cancers of most other sites, the prognosis for all patients with larynx cancer is favorable. The five-year survival rate is 64 percent. In this disease, a five-year survival is considered a cure.

The Nasal Cavity, Sinuses, and Nasopharynx

Basically, the nasal cavity is the inside of the front part of the nose. The back part of the inside of the nose, called the nasopharynx, ends where the throat begins. The sinuses are hollows within the facial

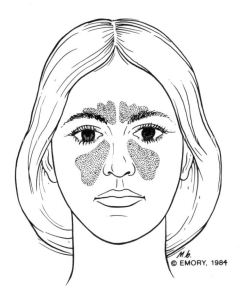

© EMORY, 1984

Shaded areas indicate sinuses

bones. The largest, the maxillary sinus, is in the cheekbone under the eye and nearly touching the roots of the upper teeth. The lining of the nasal cavity, the sinuses, and nasopharynx traps inhaled dust in the mucus produced by glands in the lining, and propels the particles backward into the throat, where they are swallowed.

Cancers in these three areas cause less than 2 percent of the cancers in the United States, or about 3,000 each year. About 60 percent of all such cancers are squamous. Adenocancers, arising from the mucus-making glands, account for 10 to 15 percent of the total. Lymphomas, arising from lymphoid tissue deposits, may also occur. Unfortunately, the symptoms for any of these cancers are nonspecific and difficult to pinpoint and are often present for several months prior to diagnosis. Nasal discharge, obstruction of air in one or both nostrils, and bleeding can be early symptoms. Cancers of the maxillary sinus are often first manifested by an aching or loosening of the upper teeth or by a swelling suggestive of a dental abscess. Since the maxillary sinus is immediately under the eye and the internal nasal cavity rises almost to the level of the eyes, there are sometimes eye-related symptoms, such as welling of tears. Earache (because of a common nerve pathway), ringing in the ear, and infection of the middle ear may also be early symptoms. Enlargement of the lymph nodes may occur on the sides of the neck along the carotid artery, or sometimes further back on the neck, closer to the nape. The usual method of diagnosis is by intraoperative biopsy. Because sinus areas are inaccessible by physical exam, regular X rays or CT (computerized tomography) scans may help.

Study of these three cancer sites has been hampered by their having been grouped with oral cancers in the past. However, even though the treatment—radiation with or without surgery—is the same, the cause is quite different. Smoking, and tobacco use in general, has no effect. Nasal cavity and sinus cancers are associated with industries involving production of much dust, such as furniture making, woodworking, and shoe manufacturing. Of course, each of these industries also involves other suspect agents besides dust, such as organic solvents (in furniture making) and dyes (in shoemaking), so even though dust seems the likely culprit, other factors may very well be involved. Nickel dust, produced in the manufacture of stainless steel, seems particularly carcinogenic. The rate of sinus and nasal cavity cancer in such workers is 800 times that of the general population. An atmosphere heavy with particles appears to cause nasal cavity and sinus cancer, but is not associated with an increased incidence of larynx or lung cancer. This may be due to the fact that large particles are trapped and removed in the nasal passages and sinuses without reaching the larynx or lungs.

Nasopharynx cancer, on the other hand, does not appear associated with dusty atmospheres, but may have a genetic or viral association. The incidence of this cancer, while less than 2 percent of total cancers diagnosed in Europe and the United States, constitutes 25 percent or more in most areas of China and Southeast Asia. In some provinces of China, such as Canton, 60 percent of all cancers originate in the nasopharynx. Studies of people in high-risk populations who have immigrated to low-risk countries are important in determining whether the disease is related to genetic or environmental factors, such as diet. In the case of nasopharynx cancer, migrant studies are inconclusive, because high-risk Chinese born in the United States, but with parents born in Canton, still have a high incidence—twenty times that of the normal United States population—though it is half that of high-risk Chinese still living in China. Genetic makeup is partly responsible. The Epstein-Barr virus has been cultured from the malignant cells in many patients with nasopharynx cancer. It is unknown whether the virus causes the cells to become malignant or whether it merely infects the cells after they become malignant, since viruses usually prefer rapidly growing cells, whether benign or malignant. Nasopharynx cancer is actually found more often among children and young adults (whose faster growing cells might be more susceptible) than most other kinds of cancer. In the high-risk Chinese populations, the incidence rate begins to rise in the fifteen- to nineteen-year-old group and reaches a plateau between thirty-five and sixty-four years, when it begins to decline.

Cancer of the nasal cavity and sinuses is usually treated by surgery to remove the bone where the cancer originated. A prosthesis, worn as part of a denture, is used to replace the bone. The overall cure rate is 40 to 45 percent, but depends greatly upon the extent of the disease at the time of diagnosis and treatment. Cancer of the nasopharynx is always treated by X-ray therapy. The five-year survival or cure rate for patients with this disease in the United States is about 30 percent.

TREATMENT

Radiation

Side effects of radiation therapy are those associated with normal tissue damage. Unfortunately, by virtue of its rapid cell turnover rate, the normal lining of the head and neck area is more prone to temporary damage. X-ray treatment is usually associated with dryness of the mouth, loss of taste, sore throat, and pain on swallowing. Since radiation decreases saliva production and changes its chemical composition, causing the saliva to become much thicker, the dryness of the mouth can be profound. Radiation therapy will probably make it necessary for the patient to brush her teeth gently with a soft toothbrush after every meal. The mouth should be rinsed often during waking hours with a salt solution to restore the normal environment of the mouth to the extent possible while X-ray treatment continues. Fluoride treatment of the teeth may be necessary to decrease risk of cavities. Dentures should be checked to confirm good fit and should be worn as little as possible.

Mouth and throat pain can be helped by medicated lozenges, gargles, and sprays that the physician will prescribe. These should be used before meals to allow the patient to eat more with less pain. Since spicy and sour foods will cause more pain, frequent small and bland meals should help. Soft, puréed, or liquid food may be necessary during the regimen of radiation treatment. Afterward, eating solid food should not cause pain.

The exterior skin of the head and neck region shows changes typical of X-ray therapy given elsewhere on the body. Signs of injury, such as redness, loss of hair, and occasionally even blistering, appear in several weeks. In general, patients with fairer skin have greater indications of damage. As the radiated skin heals, it appears tanned, and sometimes thicker and less pliable. Because of the decreased blood supply in the X-ray field, even minor injuries are apt to heal slowly.

These are all permanent changes. Measures that will alleviate discomfort include avoiding excessive heat, cold, or sunshine; and avoiding washing the area, except as a physician directs. Loose fitting clothes in the irradiated area are necessary to avoid irritation.

The permanent aftereffects of X-ray treatment in a particular field usually include hairlessness, dry mouth, and a decreased blood supply, which predisposes to slower healing after injury.

Chemotherapy

Cisplatin or CPDD (Platinol) and doxorubicin hydrochloride (Adriamycin) may produce marked shrinkage of cancer masses, but this is short-lived and the tumor mass quickly recurs in almost all cases. Research is under way to determine whether the drugs could be best used preoperatively. The side effects of both cisplatin and Adriamycin include the usual nausea and vomiting for the day afterward and depression of blood cell formation. Moreover, the possibility of kidney damage by cisplatin and cardiac damage by Adriamycin must be carefully monitored. Adriamycin causes scalp hairlessness, with regrowth occurring three to five months after the drug is discontinued.

Thyroid Cancer

The thyroid gland is a flat, butterfly-shaped organ about two inches at its greatest extent, and about one inch long. It lies in front of the airway, or trachea, just below the voice box, or larynx. Two important structures—the nerves, which work the muscles of the voice box, and the four tiny parathyroid glands, which control calcium metabolism—lie touching the back surface of the thyroid. The thyroid is the only source of two closely related hormones, triiodothyronine (T-3) and thyroxine (T-4), which affect the growth and metabolism of virtually all other cells in the body. The thyroid requires iodine for the production of these hormones and will take it up before any other organs. Triiodothyronine and thyroxine are stored in the thyroid in an inactive form until they are needed. The pituitary gland controls their activation and secretion by manufacturing its own hormone, called thyroid stimulating hormone. T-3 and T-4 cannot be released into the circulation without this pituitary hormone. Fortunately, T-3 and T-4 are of simple chemical structure and can be precisely reproduced by pharmaceutical companies in pill form. The resulting synthetic hormone can be taken orally, as opposed to other hormones, such as insulin, which must be injected. The thyroid also manufactures calcitonin, a minor hormone that influences calcium levels. However, calcitonin is so unimportant that its absence causes no problem.

An estimated 11,400 cases of thyroid cancer were diagnosed in

139

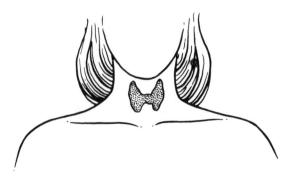

Shaded area indicates thyroid

the United States in 1984, with 7,900 in females and 3,500 in males. With 700 cancer deaths in women and 400 in men, the percentage surviving is higher among women. Thyroid cancer occurs at all ages, with three-quarters occurring in people between the ages of twenty-five and sixty-five. It is one of the more frequent malignancies of adolescence and early childhood. Thyroid cancer shows little variation country by country or region by region, and is not influenced by whether the population is agricultural or industrial, developed or undeveloped.

Thyroid cancer is designated medullary, papillary, or follicular, after its pattern of growth. An individual cancer is often a combination of the latter two microscopic pictures. Medullary cancer is responsible for about 5 to 10 percent of all thyroid cancers and arises from the C-cells that produce the hormone calcitonin. There are less than 1,000 such cases each year in the United States. Some occur among family members due to an inherited chromosomal disease and the remainder arise with no familial predisposition. Papillary refers to the malignant cells' appearing in papillae, or mounds. Follicular refers to their appearance following the natural follicle growth structure. Papillary and follicular types are responsible for 75 to 90 percent of thyroid cancers and are most commonly found in people between the ages of thirty and sixty. There is no genetic predisposition in these two kinds or in the next kind. Occurring in less than 10 percent of cases, undifferentiated, or anaplastic, cancer contains cells looking very much unlike thyroid cells. Most undifferentiated cancers occur in patients between fifty and seventy years of age.

The survival rate for patients with thyroid cancer ranges from 80 to 90 percent living over thirty years with papillary cancer to none surviving even several months the undifferentiated cancers. A United States government publication reported that of all patients with thyroid cancer, including undifferentiated, the five-year survival was 83 percent and the ten-year survival 82 percent. The five- and ten-year survival rates of those with cancer localized to the thyroid was 95 percent. Most of the time, involvement of the lymph nodes with papillary cancer, for example, does not make the individual's survival worse than if the cancer were localized to the thyroid. In either event, a 96 percent ten-year survival is the norm. In addition to so high a cure rate, the standard treatments are easy to endure compared to those for other diseases. Virtually none of the treatments interferes with childbearing.

Thyroid cancer cells are well differentiated in 80 percent of cases, meaning that, although malignant, they resemble normal thyroid cells somewhat and usually even retain some normal function.

SYMPTOMS OF THYROID CANCER

- Lump in the thyroid.
- Rarely: food sticking in mid-neck.

SYMPTOMS

In the overwhelming number of cases of thyroid cancer, the symptom leading to diagnosis is a lump found in the thyroid. This usually causes no special problem for the patient, and it is often found during a routine physical examination. Alternatively, if the lump is large enough, especially in thin women, the protruding area may be noticed by a friend or the patient herself. If the lump is large enough, perhaps two inches in diameter, it may cause symptoms because of pressure on nearby structures. For example, there may be a sticking sensation when a patient is eating solid, bulky food; it may seem to stop momentarily in the patient's midneck area while she is swallowing. Depending on its position in the neck, a large lump may cause increased pressure on the airway, accompanied by shortness of breath. Sometimes these types of discomfort are caused by a large lump located on the underside of the thyroid, which cannot be well seen or felt, but will be detected by radiologic tests.

Occasionally, with the common and easily treated thyroid cancers, the first abnormality noted is an enlarged painless lymph node, or gland, in the midneck. In other words, the actual thyroid cancer may be small and escape detection, while the lymph node enlarged by the cancer will be found first. The initial symptom of a rare undifferentiated cancer may be a hardness in the whole front area of the neck, caused by rapid spread, involving the entire gland and nearby structures.

Symptoms that have almost nothing to do with cancer are those associated with deranged thyroid metabolism, an under- or overproduction of thyroid hormone. Hyperactive thyroid (often caused by Graves' disease) may result in irritability, increased activity with insomnia, sweating, intolerance of heat, a rapid pulse rate, and weight loss despite adequate food intake. Specifically, Graves' disease is usually identified by hyperthyroid symptoms and the appearance of protruding eyes. A hypoactive thyroid causes symptoms of sluggishness, weakness, mental dullness, weight gain, and intolerance to cold. Luckily, there are accurate blood tests to determine whether such diffuse symptoms are the result of an over- or underfunctioning thyroid. Nevertheless, abnormal thyroid function is not a symptom of, and usually has nothing to do with, thyroid cancer. Thyroid hormone malfunction and thyroid cancer may sometimes be found in the same individual, but only by chance.

A diffusely enlarged thyroid, or benign goiter, which usually has many small lumps, is neither a sign nor a precursor of thyroid cancer. In the thirty- to fifty-year-old group, the incidence of benign goiter is reported to be between 4 and 8 percent.

WHO IS AT RISK?

In 1950, it became clear that even low-dose X-ray treatment of the head, neck, and upper chest—once commonly prescribed for such problems as chronic ear infections, tuberculosis, enlarged tonsils and adenoids, acne, and various other skin conditions, including fungal infections of the scalp—caused thyroid cancer, and particularly when given to children and infants. Probably because of their intense growth with rapidly dividing cells, babies more than adults, and fetuses more than babies, run an increased risk of X-ray damage. Because treatment was often administered in a dermatologist's office with small X-ray machines, the event might not be as readily remembered as X rays given by a large hospital machine. X-ray treatment for benign diseases was generally abandoned by 1960.

Studies indicate that the risk of thyroid cancer increases as the X-ray dose approaches 2,000 rads. After that, higher doses do not cause thyroid cancer—probably because the higher doses kill the thyroid cells. The lower doses are thought to damage the chromosomes while leaving the cells alive and able to reproduce themselves. As with other radiation-induced cancers, the interval between X ray and cancer production was usually one or two decades. One study found the average interval to be twenty-seven years. However, it is possible that even more cancers will be found as patients are followed longer, and that the average interval will increase.

Of those irradiated, younger children and females appear to be at greater risk. Interestingly, X ray to the thyroid more often caused benign abnormalities than cancer. In a large study of more than 1,000 patients, abnormalities were found in 27 percent of those tested. Only 7 percent were found to have cancer at the time of the test, though the true incidence is likely to rise as more patients undergo thyroid surgery for diagnosis.

Though medullary thyroid cancer arises because of a chromosomal error, many cases develop spontaneously with no familial tendency. In the chromosomal medullary disease, tumors of the adrenal and parathyroid glands also frequently occur.

Preventive Measures

In preventing thyroid cancer, it might be valuable to shield the thyroid, especially in children and adolescents, during routine diagnostic X rays. A lead apron should be used during dental X rays. Unfortunately, the neck area cannot be shielded in chest X rays without also obscuring the top of the chest. However, since the dose of a chest X ray is less than 1/1,000 of the typical dose that would cause thyroid cancer, the diagnostic benefits far outweigh the risks of thyroid cancer.

DIAGNOSIS

According to various reports, a single lump or nodule is found during the physical examination of the thyroid in 1 to 7 percent of the healthy American population. In a typical series of patients who underwent removal of the thyroid for a solitary lump, cancer was found in only 18 percent. Nodules are less common in men, though a higher proportion of them are cancer. Nodules, while more common in women, are somewhat less likely to be malignant.

Because of the high incidence of thyroid lumps and the relative low occurrence of cancer, accurate diagnosis before an operation is important in order to avoid unnecessary surgery on benign lumps. Worrisome factors include a history of radiation therapy, a relatively recent onset of a hard single nodule, and, of course, the presence of enlarged neck lymph nodes. The various methods of diagnosis involve suppression of the function of the thyroid gland, the use of ultrasound scanning with radioactive isotopes, and aspiration by needle.

Thyroid Gland Suppression

Suppression of the thyroid gland is accomplished by the use of thyroid hormone replacement pills for two to three months or longer. The pituitary responds to this treatment by ceasing production of a particular pituitary hormone, without which the thyroid will not produce its hormones. The whole thyroid gland, including the enlarged nodules, will thus become dormant and diminish in size. Since cancerous nodules are much less sensitive to normal pituitary control than are benign nodules, the malignant nodules should be unaffected while the benign nodules should shrink. In practice, though, less than half the benign nodules shrink and disappear with this test. Moreover, a thyroid cancer nodule, if composed of papillary or follicular cancer, will occasionally shrink somewhat, since these common cancers somewhat resemble normal tissue. Therefore, the test can be misleading.

Ultrasound

The thyroid can also be evaluated by the use of reflected sound waves. Harmless high-frequency sound waves penetrate the thyroid and bounce back at various rates depending on the density of the tissue. The reflected sound waves are picked up by a sensor and are graphically displayed, forming an image of the thyroid gland. The exam is usually performed in the X-ray department of a hospital or clinic, with the patient lying on her back. A gel is applied to the patient's neck to facilitate movement of the sound source and sensor over that area. Breathing and swallowing are not hindered during the test. Because X rays are not used and there are no complications or discomfort, the exam is safe and may be repeated as necessary. Ultrasound is valuable for distinguishing a cyst, which is fluid-filled, from a solid lump. (Cysts are malignant only about 1 percent of the time and can be removed by needle drainage without surgery.) In addition, because of the superficial position of the thyroid in the body, lumps as small as half an inch should be visible with ultrasound.

Thyroid Scan

A thyroid scan can often determine the size, shape, position, and functional abnormalities of a lump in the thyroid gland. A radioactive substance, such as iodine or technetium, is given by mouth. After a suitable time, a scanning camera is placed over the neck and a record, in the form of a photograph or X ray of the radiation emitted by various areas of the thyroid, is produced. If the areas do not take up the iodine or technetium, nodules are classified as "cold" and may be benign tumors, cysts, or cancers. Nodules are "hot" if they take up more radioactive substance than the surrounding thyroid tissue. Only about 1 percent of hot nodules are cancers; almost all are benign tumors, called adenomas. Because this test shows the general outline of the thyroid, it can often determine whether a lump in the neck actually arises from the thyroid gland or from another structure nearby. Recent radioactive studies, even X-ray dye studies, may interfere with this test. Pregnant women, in general, should never be given radioactive substances.

Technetium is a safer substance, since radioactive iodine may be associated with a low incidence of radiation-induced cancer. But, in order to measure the thyroid's function, as is necessary in suspected under- or overfunctioning of the thyroid, radioactive iodine must be used. The uptake rate of iodine—an essential component of thyroid hormone—is measured by scan at regular intervals after its administration. However, this part of the test is not necessary for mere diagnosis of a nodule.

Needle Aspiration of the Nodule

Aspiration of a thyroid nodule by needle and syringe is a simple and safe technique performed by those experienced in its usage—usually surgeons and some endocrinologists who know the anatomy of the neck in detail. A needle of the size used for drawing blood is inserted into the nodule. If the nodule is a cyst, the fluid contents will be drawn out and may then be sent for microscopic analysis. Only 1 or 2 percent of cysts with clear fluid contain cancer, with the percentage increasing if the fluid is bloody. If the nodule is a solid lump, the aspiration will draw forth a small number of cells that can be microscopically analyzed. A recent study by a cancer center proficient in this technique has found that an adequate number of cells could be obtained from 90 percent of the nodules. Only rarely did cases diagnosed as cancer turn out to be benign on microscopic analysis after thyroid removal. By the same token, only 5 to 10 percent of the nodules diagnosed as benign by needle aspiration later proved to be cancer upon thyroid removal. As with any needle technique, it is possible to unknowingly gather benign cells adjacent to a malignant nodule. Accordingly, anyone who does not undergo surgery for a thyroid nodule diagnosed as benign by needle aspiration must undergo careful follow-up exam, since the nodule may actually be cancerous.

Sequence of Tests

Since surgery for benign nodules is to be avoided when possible, a number of test sequences are followed. I might try aspiration of the nodule at the first visit. If the nodule is a cyst and the fluid is diagnosed benign by microscopic analysis, one visit solves the problem. However, according to various studies, only 10 to 25 percent of nodules are actually cysts. If the microscopic analysis shows malignant cells, the patient would be prepared for surgery. If the microscopic analysis shows benign cells, I would continue diagnostic tests for the possibility that the nodule was still a cancer, but that the needle missed the malignant cells. This sequence might then include ultrasound, thyroid scan, and thyroid suppression. Depending on the test results, surgery might also be recommended.

TREATMENT

Surgery

The initial treatment of thyroid cancer is surgery, with the infrequent exception of rare, undifferentiated cancers (in which case two factors often preclude surgery: early invasion of essential neck structures and early distant spread to lungs, liver, etc.). The standard operation is removal of all or part of the thyroid gland with the patient under general anesthesia, and the procedure itself takes about three hours. The incision, basic for all thyroidectomies, is three and a half or four inches long and is placed symmetrically horizontal and significantly lower in the neck than the actual thyroid. Since the normal wrinkling of the neck skin is also horizontal, the incision heals in a fine line resembling a wrinkle. Since there is little or no tension in this area, the scar does not have a tendency to widen, as do scars on the abdomen, for example. Because the blood supply of the neck is better than that of the abdomen or limbs, healing is faster, allowing the stitches to be removed quite early, usually in two to four days, and to be replaced with strips of surgical tape. Early removal should also prevent tiny, circular, stitch-hole scars on either side of the incision. It is always possible to hide the incision in the lower neck with a blouse collar, though few find cover-up necessary. Usually, the lobe, or half of the thyroid, is removed and sent for frozen section and microscopic analysis while the patient is still asleep. Some patients have asked why the lump alone cannot be removed for frozen section, with the remainder of the lobe left. Were the lump diagnosed as benign— as it usually is—no thyroid replacement therapy would then be necessary. This is not done because operating on a particular lobe produces enough scarring around the parathyroids and nerves to make reoperation upon those structures quite dangerous. Therefore, the entire thyroid lobe is removed at the first operation. A lobectomy is appropriate surgical treatment because frozen section analysis of thyroid tissue is not completely accurate. Were the thyroid lump found benign upon examination of cells from an intraoperative frozen section, but later proven malignant upon examination of the samples prepared for permanent pathology, there would be no reason to reoperate if the entire lobe had been removed. If another lump were to develop in the remainder of the operated-upon lobe, it could present a higher complication rate for reoperation than would the original operation, because of scarring. Blood tests reveal that many patients can do without oral thyroid replacement after lobe removal. On the other hand, most doctors do recommend that patients take an oral thyroid replacement to make the thyroid inactive, thereby minimizing the chances of developing a new nodule, benign or malignant.

If the frozen section reveals papillary cancer, controversy exists as to whether an adequate operation consists of removal of the lobe (about half of the thyroid) or of subtotal removal of the entire thyroid gland (80 to 85 percent of the gland). Proponents of the more extensive operation point out that microscopically found cancer cells may exist in the opposite lobe in 30 percent or more of patients with papillary cancer. Proponents of the less extensive surgery argue that microscopic deposits mean nothing. They note that survival rates are similar for both procedures, but that the complication rate—due to damage to the parathyroid and larynx (voice box)—is much higher for the more extensive procedure.

If the frozen section determines follicular cancer, the same arguments apply. In addition, with this type of thyroid cancer, many doctors argue for a total removal (95 to 100 percent of the gland), which has an even higher complication rate. With complete thyroid removal, the diagnosis and treatment of the spread of follicular cancer, and sometimes, of papillary cancer, will be simpler.

If the frozen section determines medullary cancer, a total thyroid removal, sometimes with removal of the neck lymph nodes, is the preferred procedure. About half these patients have obviously enlarged lymph nodes that must also be removed at the time of diagnosis. This cancer is more aggressive than papillary and follicular, though less so than the undifferentiated, and only half of all patients with medullary cancer are cured.

Recovery from a thyroid removal is usually rapid and relatively painless compared to recovery from chest or abdominal operations. The patient can drink and even eat on the night of her surgery. A soft drain, acting like a wick, may be left in place for a day or two to handle any residual oozing. The patient is usually discharged on the fourth postoperative day. The neck will be sore and the voice hoarse for about a week. If there are any complications, the voice may be hoarse for a longer term.

As mentioned previously, the parathyroid glands lie on the underside of the thyroid, one near each of the four corners. The hormone they produce, called parathormone, controls the metabolism of calcium, one of the most important minerals required by the body. Calcium controls the contraction of all muscle, whether cardiac or limb, and the conduction in the nerves. Because of their small size (a quarter of an inch), their indistinguishable color, and their adherence to the thyroid, the parathyroids are prone to injury if all four areas of the thyroid are dissected, as is done in a total thyroidectomy or, occasionally, in a subtotal thyroidectomy. However, if two or even three parathyroids are injured, the body can still function normally with only one gland. Permanent lack of parathormone due to injury of all four glands occurs in about 10 percent of cases of total thyroid removal. If this happens, calcium metabolism can be regulated—although with difficulty—by oral medication taken several times a day, accompanied by careful blood monitoring. When the injury is recognized at the operation, recent research has shown that injured parathyroids can be transplanted into neck muscle, where they will heal and function normally. Therefore, as time goes on, the number of patients with no parathyroid function may decrease due to transplantation.

Another complication of thyroidectomies involves damage to one or both nerves that control the voice box. With only one side of the thyroid dissected, there exists the possibility of damage to only one nerve; with both sides, to both nerves. If one nerve is damaged, the voice will become immediately hoarse and will tire after brief intervals of speaking. After several weeks, the nonparalyzed nerve will have increased its strength to the point where hoarseness will usually be absent. However, if both nerves are paralyzed, the consequences are worse, often resulting in a permanent tracheostomy. The incidence of damage to both vocal cord nerves is less than 1 percent in total thyroidectomies.

Radiation

External beam radiation therapy is rarely used to shrink malignant growths, because radioactive iodine is a much more effective means for utilizing X ray on the thyroid.

Normal thyroid tissue attracts and concentrates iodine to the exclusion of all other tissues in the body. Therefore, when radioactive iodine is administered, it is taken up by the thyroid, destroying normal tissue. Because papillary and follicular cancers retain some normal thyroid function, they also usually take up iodine, although to a smaller extent than normal tissue. For this reason, papillary and follicular cancers attract radioactive iodine and are destroyed by it. (Medullary and undifferentiated cancers do not act like normal thyroid tissue and do not take up iodine.) While the radioactive isotope is strong and the radiation dosage to the thyroid itself is much higher than that which can be administered by external beam, the radiation penetrates only a short distance. In practice, only the tissue that takes up the radioactive iodine will be destroyed by it. This is true not only for papillary and follicular cancers in the neck, but also for the rare instances in which they have spread to other organs, such as the lung, liver, bone, etc. If tumor-seeking radioactive elements could be devised for other malignancies, cancer therapy would be greatly simplified.

The radioactive iodine is administered by swallowing a liquid. The complications of radioactive iodine therapy include nausea, vomiting, and depressed platelet and white blood cell counts. These side effects, however, are not as marked as those from chemotherapy. Moreover, they are present only with actual iodine administration, which is usually necessary only once.

Thyroid Hormone Therapy

Added to other therapies for papillary and follicular cancers, long-term thyroid hormone administration by pill improves the cure rate, and does so without side effects. Thyroid stimulating hormone, produced by the pituitary gland, promotes the growth and division of papillary and follicular cancers to a greater or lesser extent in various individuals; therefore, oral hormone replacement is almost always recommended in doses large enough to suppress its production—usually 0.15 mg to 0.3 mg of thyroxine. The actual dosage necessary for hormone suppression can be determined by testing blood samples for the virtual disappearance of thyroid stimulating hormone.

Chemotherapy

Chemotherapy is only rarely used for thyroid cancer. Not many patients require it, as the disease is easily curable or treatable by other means. In the case of undifferentiated cancers, doxorubicin hydrochloride (Adriamycin) has been used most frequently with the same side effects as in breast or ovarian cancer, where it is used more frequently. The common side effects include nausea, vomiting, hairlessness, depressed blood cell counts, and heart damage at higher doses.

Esophageal Cancer

C ancer of the esophagus is one of the less common gastrointestinal malignancies. There were an estimated 9,000 cases diagnosed in the United States in 1984 compared to 130,000 cases of colon and rectal cancer. Seventy percent of all esophageal cancer is diagnosed in men, 30 percent in women, but worldwide the sex ratio is more equal. Like other gastrointestinal cancers, cancer of the esophagus arises from the cells lining that organ.

The esophagus, the passageway for food between the throat and the stomach, passes from the neck, through the chest, and into the abdomen. A muscular tube, it begins at the larynx, or voice box, where the common air and food passageway separates into the trachea, or main airway, to the lungs and into the esophagus. The esophagus is about an inch and a half in diameter when empty and stretches as food passes through. The swallowing reflex causes the esophageal muscle to contract involuntarily in a wavelike fashion, pushing the food down toward the stomach.

The esophagus extends downward adjacent to the spine, the aorta (the largest blood vessel in the body), and the trachea for much of its length. In addition, the esophagus is very close to the neck arteries leading to the brain, the lung, the diaphragm, and the back wall of the heart.

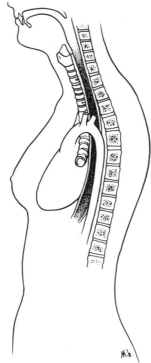

Shaded area indicates esophagus

SYMPTOMS OF ESOPHAGEAL CANCER

- Difficulty swallowing.
- Sensation of food sticking in neck or chest.

SYMPTOMS

The most easily recognized symptom of esophageal cancer is difficulty in swallowing and a sensation of food sticking due to obstruction by the malignant growth. Foods that typically cause this are meats; "rough" fruits, such as apples; and fresh, nontoasted bread, which forms lumps of dough when swallowed. These foods tend to catch momentarily on the esophagus cancer, causing a sticking sensation that usually passes within several minutes.

Unfortunately, when difficulty in swallowing occurs, a patient may merely eliminate the troublesome foods from the diet rather than see a doctor. As long as such foods are avoided, the swallowing appears to have returned to normal. If the symptoms have been caused by a cancer, however, the tumor will continue to grow undiagnosed, and within a matter of time, perhaps several months, other, less bulky foods will cause the same difficulty. If these symptoms are ignored, even softer and more liquid foods will eventually produce difficulty in swallowing, and the patient will reach the point when only fluids can be swallowed. In the meantime, the golden opportunity for early detection and simple treatment will have been lost. *Symptoms should never be ignored.* If a particular doctor does not take your symptoms seriously, find one who will.

WHO IS AT RISK?

There is no genetic or familial predisposition to esophageal cancer. However, the incidence increases with age, both in the high- and low-risk areas.

Geographical Factors

Even though it is relatively uncommon in the United States, esophageal cancer is a leading cause of death in some parts of China, Asiatic Russia, and Iran. In those particular areas, it may occur with a frequency rate ten times that of any other cancer.

Esophageal cancer also exhibits a very peculiar characteristic: It has a tremendous swing of occurrence and death rate over short geographic distances. While the rate in one of the so-called hot spots is very high, a hundred miles away it can be very low. Linxian Province, in China, is one such hot spot; the province immediately adjacent to it has a low rate, similar to that of the United States. Public health experts feel that this pattern indicates an external or environmental cancer-causing agent in the high-incidence areas. Intensive research has sometimes succeeded in identifying the particular carcinogen, which often proves to be dietary. In Linxian Province, for example, researchers noted that backyard chickens often developed cancer of the swallowing mechanism. The human cancer was traced back to this observation: pickled vegetable scraps caused an esophageal-like cancer in the chickens. The inhabitants of the province consume large amounts of the pickled vegetables as a favorite relish. It is still unknown, however, whether the apparent carcinogenic nature of the vegetables is due to the acidity, the coarseness, or possibly even to chemical contamination.

Poverty

Whether in hot spots or areas of low incidence, esophageal cancer is associated with poorer socioeconomic classes. In a ten-city survey conducted in the United States, those classified as poorest have at least two-and-a-half times the esophageal cancer of the wealthiest, even after other known risk factors, such as smoking, are taken into account. It is not known what is responsible for this rich/poor difference. Although one might imagine that the poor would have more of every type of cancer than the rich, this is not the case; in fact, some cancers occur more often in the wealthy. Nutritional differences may be significant, though this theory has not been proven.

Smoking and Alcohol Consumption

Habitual intake of alcohol and tobacco has always been associated with esophageal cancer. In North America and Western Europe, it is estimated that up to 90 percent of people with esophageal cancer are tobacco smokers (whether of cigarettes, pipes, or cigars) and daily users of alcohol. In the late sixties, a study was conducted involving 68,000 men in labor unions who were identified as cigarette smokers or nonsmokers. These men were followed for several years to record their various illnesses and causes of death. Not surprisingly, cancer of the esophagus was one of the four cancers found in significantly higher rates in smokers than nonsmokers. (The other smoker-associated cancers were lung, bladder, and mouth, throat, and larynx.)

However, in some high-frequency areas, such as Linxian Province, use of alcohol and tobacco is uncommon. And in the northern Gonbad region of Iran, while consumption of alcohol and cigarette smoking is also rare, there is a local practice of eating the opium residue left in the pipe. This practice is strongly associated with the risk of esophageal cancer. Also, this practice is found only in the lowest socioeconomic classes—those who are unemployed and live in poverty, like the addicts of any society. No studies have been done as yet on the effects of marijuana smoking.

Evidence suggests that consumption of wine and beer by itself does not necessarily increase the risk of esophageal cancer, but consumption of concentrated alcohol, such as gin, vodka, and whiskey, does increase the risks significantly. Alcohol and tobacco working together produce a combined risk of esophageal cancer significantly greater than the sum of the two taken separately. That is, were the risk associated with the use of alcohol equal to X percent and that of tobacco equal to Y percent, the risk to a person using both would not be X *plus* Y percent but closer to X *times* Y percent.

Tobacco smoke, with its many separate cancer-causing chemicals, condenses in the saliva and is physically in contact, as a thin film, with the cells lining the esophagus. Alcohol may act as a solvent on the carcinogens, allowing them to dissolve more completely. The carcinogens could then better penetrate the outer lining cells of the esophagus and harm the vulnerable dividing cells of the inner lining.

Alcohol also has a drying effect, as can be seen when cosmetic preparations containing alcohol cause chapping and cracking of the skin. A similar drying effect may injure the esophagus lining and predispose the damaged cells to more rapid action by whatever carcinogens come into contact with them. This may be why the drinking of wine, which has a lower alcohol content, is a smaller risk factor for esophageal cancer than the drinking of concentrated alcohol.

Other Risk Factors

A condition called Barrett's lining, involving abnormal but benign cells growing in the lower or middle esophagus, predisposes to cancer. Another predisposing condition is achalasia, in which the sphincter muscle of the lowermost esophagus does not relax well, blocking the easy passage of food.

Almost all substances are more soluble in hot liquids than in cold, which may explain why hot food in general is associated with esophageal cancer in some of the hot spot areas. The other effect of the high temperature might be similar to that of the drying effects of alcohol: heat injures cells upon direct contact, thereby making it easier for carcinogens to penetrate.

Of the approximately 5,000 children each year who drink lye or other caustic liquids, the ones who survive are prone to high esophageal cancer rates as adults. In one group followed for twenty-four years, the rate of occurrence for such people was 1,000 times the expected rate in the normal population.

Data from atomic bomb survivors at Hiroshima and Nagasaki, and from patients with spinal disease who were treated with X rays, show somewhat higher than normal rates of esophageal cancer. This is not surprising, since, like most tissue, the esophagus is susceptible to the effects of radiation.

In the United States, the highest rate of esophageal cancer is found in the southeast; the reasons are unknown. Statistically, blacks are affected more than whites. Even though black males constitute only about 6 percent of the American population, they account for 18 percent of the disease.

DETECTION AND DIAGNOSIS

Diagnosis of esophageal cancer depends upon visualization of the malignancy either indirectly with an X ray or directly with a "see-through" flexible tube used to examine the lining of the structure itself. In the United States and other countries where the rate of esophageal cancer is quite low, hundreds of thousands of individuals without symptoms would have to be tested to find a single case. The disease is relatively uncommon, even among those of the higher risk categories mentioned earlier.

In some hot spot areas, there are public health programs promoting routine screening tests for this cancer on people without any symptoms, just as American physicians encourage routine Pap smears. In these areas, the screening programs are cost effective because so many patients are diagnosed at an early stage. Early diagnosis of a small cancer means the curative treatment can be simple, and, of course, less costly in the end.

In China, the government sends mobile vans (much like the chest X-ray vans used in the 1950s in the United States) into hot spots so that nurses and technicians can administer a quick and efficient test for esophageal cancer. The test involves the swallowing of a very thin tube with the diameter and flexibility of string. At the end of the tube is a collapsed balloon covered by a nylon net. Once the balloon is in the stomach, it is blown up to the size of a dime and then pulled out through the esophagus and mouth. As it travels from bottom to top, the abrasive action of the balloon's nylon net collects samples of the lining cells. These cells are then wiped onto microscope slides (similar to the process in a Pap smear) and studied under the microscope. If the slides show malignant cells, further tests and subsequent treatment are required.

Barium Swallow

Another diagnostic procedure, the barium swallow, involves the X-ray dye barium; a radiologist watches its progress on a fluoroscopy machine and/or records it on movie films. As the barium is swallowed, its passage along the whole esophagus is observed and any blockage is noted. In addition, the barium outlines the esophageal lining during and after its passage and will show the narrower or otherwise abnormal spots. If the thick liquid barium does not show any problem, a barium "burger" may be tried. In this test, the patient swallows a barium-coated hamburger or barium-coated bread to allow the radiologist a visualization of where the dye-covered food slows or stops. As you can imagine, however, not everything can be accurately seen on an X ray and often endoscopy is required.

Endoscopy

In this test a flexible lighted tube about the width of a thick ballpoint pen is swallowed under local anesthesia. The equipment's special lens and magnification allow the physician to thoroughly examine every square inch of the esophageal lining. Because esophageal cancer always starts on the surface lining, this is an ideal test, and it can detect the disease with close to 100 percent accuracy. Endoscopy is costly and uncomfortable and has a small (less than 1 percent) complication rate, so it is used only when the expectation of finding an esophagus abnormality justifies the risk.

TREATMENT

Surgery

Esophageal cancer has a lower cure rate than many other gastrointestinal cancers—only about 5 percent. This probably results from the peculiar anatomy of the esophagus and the tendency of this cancer to spread quickly to important organs. However, if it is found early, cancer of the esophagus can be operated upon with generally good results. Since the esophagus lies adjacent to the spine, the main airway, and the body's largest blood vessel, any esophagus operation—particularly an operation to remove it—is a significant undertaking. For these reasons, the operation has a high complication rate and carries a greater risk of death than most others. Some older patients, whose medical condition is satisfactory for other kinds of surgery, may not be able to tolerate an esophagus operation.

The operation itself may be performed from a chest incision, an abdominal incision, or even a neck incision, depending upon the cancer's precise location. The procedure involves removal of the esophagus and its replacement with some kind of natural tube as a passageway for food. Unfortunately, despite great advances in organ replacement, no suitable synthetic tube has yet been found that can be used to replace the esophagus. While the arterial wall heals into the "cloth" tubes used to replace blocked arteries, and the synthetic grafts behave quite like normal tissue, the esophagus will not heal to anything but other parts of the gastrointestinal tract. Accordingly, the operation consists, in part, of bringing into the chest a portion of the gastrointestinal tract to act as the passageway, and of sewing it to the remaining two ends. In the past, the stomach, small bowel, and large bowel have all been used for this purpose.

Most surgeons prefer to use the stomach, which, when surgically loosened from all of its surrounding structures, can be led all the way through the chest into the neck. This procedure usually involves less surgery than using other organs for the replacement. The Chinese, who have the most cases of esophageal cancer, also use the stomach. However, previous or current stomach disease, such as an ulcer, may mean the stomach is not loose enough to reach into the chest, and therefore cannot be used. In that case, the colon is often used, though some surgeons prefer to use the colon in the first place. Operations for esophageal cancer are relatively infrequent, and surgeons tend to become expert in one technique above others. When part of the colon is removed for esophagus replacement, the remaining ends of the colon are joined back together so that bowel movement follows its normal path, and a colostomy is unnecessary.

The main problem peculiar to esophageal cancer, as you can see, is the swallowing mechanism; patients with advanced disease are unable to swallow even liquids. When the disease is critically advanced, they cannot swallow their own saliva and have to spit or drool to be rid of it. These patients can be fed liquids through a tube placed into the stomach and exiting through the skin of the abdomen. This procedure is strictly functional, since taste is impossible. Also, the saliva problem still remains.

A variety of plastic and metal tubes have been created for placement down the esophagus and through the cancer to allow food to pass from the mouth to the stomach—though only food in the form of thick liquids will pass well. These tubes can often be placed with the same flexible lighted scope that is used for diagnosis. But when this simple procedure does not work, the patient requires surgery under general anesthesia for placement of a tube directly into the stomach through an abdominal incision.

Radiation

Aside from an inadequate physical condition, some patients cannot undergo the operation because their cancer is too advanced to be cured. They are often treated by X-ray therapy, which may hold the tumor in check and keep its growth at a plateau for several months. Though patients are occasionally cured by radiation therapy, surgery is usually more successful and is the first choice in good-risk patients.

Chemotherapy

Drugs are usually employed only to treat the spread of this cancer to distant organs. Bleomycin (Blenoxane), cisplatin (Platinol), and 5-FU Fluorouracil/mitomycin (Mutamycin) combinations have a significant remission rate.

Pancreatic Cancer

The pancreas is a thin, flat organ perhaps twelve inches in length and three inches at the point of greatest width. It lies behind the other organs of the upper abdomen, running from the liver on the right to the spleen on the left, crossing the spinal column. The pancreas will not appear on barium X-ray tests designed to outline the gastrointestinal tract. Since the organ is surrounded by tissues of much the same consistency as the pancreas itself, there is even difficulty visualizing it by ultrasonography and CT scan, though these tests are still the most useful. The pancreas serves two functions. First, it produces digestive juices, or enzymes, that break down carbohydrates, proteins, and fats. Abnormalities or inflammation of the pancreas, often resulting from excess alcohol, hinder the body's absorption of fats in particular. The second function of the pancreas involves the production of various hormones, the most important of which is insulin. Accordingly, pancreatic diseases can cause diabetes mellitus, or sugar diabetes. In the greatest majority of cases, however, diabetes is *not* caused by cancer.

Cancer of the pancreas is the fifth-greatest cause of cancer-related deaths each year in the United States after cancers of the lung, colon, breast, and prostate. Overall, there is a 1.1 percent chance of developing this cancer, which strikes twice as many men as women. Rare before the age of forty, most cases occur in the seventh and eighth

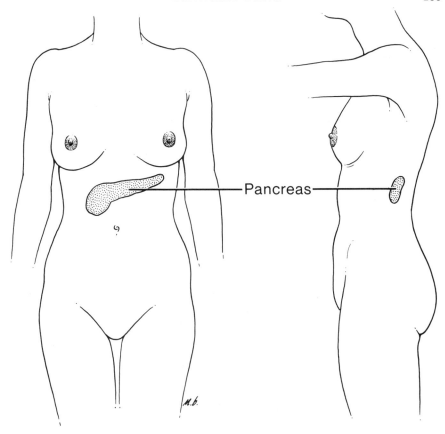

Front and side views of pancreas

decades of life. Unfortunately, cancer of the pancreas has one of the lowest cure rates. Less than 5 percent of people diagnosed with the disease will survive five years. In more than 90 percent of pancreas cancers, the point of origin is the cells that line the ducts which transport the digestive enzymes to the intestines. In a small percentage of cases, the cell of origin may be that actually producing the hormones.

SYMPTOMS OF PANCREATIC CANCER

- Vague sensations of ill health, sometimes indigestion.
- Yellowing of skin and eyes.
- Pain, usually above the navel, often radiating around like a belt or straight through to the back.
- Infrequently: invisible blood mixed into the bowel movement.

SYMPTOMS

Pancreatic cancer is rarely diagnosed early enough to allow for curative surgery. The earliest stages produce no symptoms, and when symptoms do begin, they are often intermittent for several days or weeks before they become constant. Furthermore, though the person may have had symptoms for several months prior to diagnosis, the symptoms tend to be so nonspecific as to indicate little of their true cause. A patient may complain of a vague sensation of ill health, loss of weight, irregularity of bowel movements, and sometimes what may simply be called indigestion, before clearer symptoms appear. And as the pancreas is adjacent to other organs in the upper abdomen, the symptoms sometimes appear associated with those organs instead of with the pancreas.

The symptoms of pancreatic cancer depend to some extent upon the part of the gland in which the cancer originates. In three-quarters of the cases, the cancer arises in the head of the organ on the right side. If this is the case, the cancerous mass may block the duct that carries bile from the liver to the intestines. Bile then seeps back into the bloodstream, causing the yellowing of the skin and eyes known as jaundice. Bile also passes into the urine, which becomes brownish in color. Since the bile is prevented from reaching the digestive system, the stool, normally dark-brown in color, may be pale gray or beige.

Pain is a symptom of all forms of pancreatic cancer, particularly when the cancer arises in the middle of the organ. Usually felt just above the navel, sometimes radiating around the body like a belt, pain can come and go in an irregular fashion. Because the middle of the pancreas rests on the spine, a tumor can produce a boring sensation radiating toward the center of the back. The pain is often worse at night and is eased by sitting up and bending forward. Because the pancreas lies behind the stomach, a doctor may falsely suspect that the pain of pancreatic cancer is caused by an ulcer.

Occasionally, blood from the pancreatic cancer will pass painlessly through the pancreatic duct into the intestine. This will cause a low blood count, and blood will be found when the stool is tested. Because of the proximity of the gallbladder, pain originating in the pancreas is occasionally blamed on gallstones, and the cancer is found only when the gallbladder is removed.

There are other symptoms that, while more likely to be the result of noncancerous causes, would lead to the diagnostic tests for pancreatic cancer. One is the appearance of diabetes mellitus, or sugar diabetes, especially if the disease is not present in other family members, or is not prompted by a condition such as obesity. Another is unexplained weight loss. In this case, a person may be pleased to lose weight without the usual difficult dieting, but then becomes alarmed as the weight loss continues uncontrolled. Weight loss without dieting should always be a signal for a checkup. In pancreatic cancer, weight loss can result from decreased appetite, nausea or vomiting, mental depression from pain, or loss of pancreatic enzymes, so that food is poorly digested and valuable nutrients lost. A third possibility, already mentioned, is persistent ulcer symptoms. Ulcers are frequently and sometimes falsely blamed for any upper abdominal symptom, since about 10 percent of the American population will have a stomach or duodenal ulcer at some point in their lifetime. Usually, the patient thinks the vague symptoms are the result of exercise, overwork, or stress, and that they will be relieved by resting or applying heat. She or he is reassured because the symptoms come and go. Only when the symptoms persist over time is the individual likely to visit a physician. When the discomfort is described, it may be so unlocalized as to suggest no particular diagnosis, and a nonspecific medicine, such as antacids, may be recommended at first.

WHO IS AT RISK?

Over the past fifty years, there has been a gradual three- to fourfold increase in the incidence of pancreatic cancer in the United States, with similar increases in Japan, Great Britain, and other developed countries. Four decades ago, there were only 5,000 cases reported in the United States annually; but in 1983, there were an estimated 22,000. While the population has increased and people are living longer, these factors have been accounted for. The increasing incidence also appears to have leveled off in the past several years. Some researchers believe the occurrence of pancreatic cancer has not risen, instead they feel that doctors are just accurately diagnosing it more often. In past decades, without modern tests, elderly patients thought to have died of "old age" may have died from cancer of the pancreas.

The difference in incidence of pancreatic cancer from country to country is one of the smallest for all cancers. Since it is precisely the difference in rates between various countries that often provides clues as to specific causes, the fact that most countries have almost the same amount of pancreatic cancer suggests that it is caused by a combination of widespread, generalized factors.

Diabetes

It is doubtful that diabetes—a common disease of the pancreas—is related to the cause of pancreatic cancer. On the other hand, cancer of the pancreas can cause diabetes by extensively affecting the pancreatic cells that produce insulin. Sometimes diabetes is so mild that it produces no typical symptoms—such as excess urination, excessive thirst, and fatigue—and can be detected only through a glucose tolerance test. In this test, the patient drinks a high-sugar solution and has blood drawn at frequent intervals thereafter to determine whether the pancreas can handle the increased sugar.

Whether long-standing diabetes predisposes someone to pancreatic cancer can be studied by evaluating the kinds of diseases causing death in diabetics. One study compared the cause of death in 21,000 diabetics with the cause of death in nondiabetics. The results showed that diabetics experience only a slightly higher death rate from pancreatic cancer than nondiabetics. The large number of people studied probably allowed this slight difference to emerge, where smaller studies revealed no difference at all. Accordingly, diabetes does not significantly predispose to cancer of the pancreas.

Pancreas Inflammation

The development of pancreatic cancer and prior inflammation of the pancreas appear related. In particular, many investigators believe that long-term excessive alcohol intake—the most common cause of pancreas inflammation—may be related to the development of pancreas cancer. Gallstones can also cause irritation or inflammation of the pancreas when they leave the gallbladder and pass through the duct in the midst of the pancreas; some researchers have noted a slight association between gallstones and pancreatic cancer.

Coffee Consumption

A recent study by the Harvard School of Public Health has suggested that coffee intake is related to an increased incidence of pancreatic cancer and that tea consumption is not. Decaffeinated and regular coffee consumption were not analyzed separately.

If the risk of consuming no coffee were accepted as baseline, women who drink one to two cups of coffee daily have 2.1 times the risk of women who never drink coffee. Consuming three to four cups caused 2.8 times the risk, and five or more cups, 3.2 times the risk. The results of this study are as yet uncorroborated and will need further evaluation from other centers. Criticism of the research has focused on the fact that the relative risks were derived by comparing the coffee-drinking habits of other hospitalized patients with those of pancreatic cancer patients. Patients hospitalized for gastrointestinal diseases, such as ulcers, probably would not drink coffee—precisely *because* of their ulcers. The same may be true for patients with various other diseases resulting in hospitalization. Accordingly, though pancreatic cancer patients may drink no more than the average American, they may very well drink more coffee than other hospitalized patients. This would result in the impression that coffee causes cancer of the pancreas.

I do not mean to imply that coffee is harmless. I mean only to suggest that there is no definite evidence of its causing pancreatic cancer. In fact, one researcher suggests that the chlorogenic acid in coffee may produce the carcinogenic nitrosamines from nitrites normally present in the diet. In addition, the extra steps in the chemical processing of decaffeinated coffee may themselves be factors that require further investigation.

The Cigarette Factor

Research studies following cigarette smokers over a period of years in the United States, Canada, and Japan show that smokers have twice the risk of developing cancer of the pancreas as nonsmokers. This increased risk for smokers is, however, significantly less than their risk of developing the smoking-related malignancies of the lung, throat, bladder, and esophagus. Ex-smokers also have higher risk of pancreatic cancer, though clearly not as high as that of current smokers. Smoking habits would also seem to explain the fact that twice as many men have pancreatic cancer as women; the incidence of pancreas cancer appears not to differ much among nonsmoking women and nonsmoking men.

The risk does not rise significantly with the number of cigarettes smoked: one pack of cigarettes per day is as dangerous as three packs. This may seem surprising, but heavy smokers have such high death rates from lung cancer, other lung diseases, and heart diseases that they may not live long enough to develop pancreatic cancer. The data on cigarette smoking and its association with a twofold increase in pancreas cancer are consistent and repeatable, and derive from more than twenty reliable studies. Cigar and pipe smokers also appear to be at increased risk from cancer of the pancreas, suggesting that the specific carcinogen is absorbed into the bloodstream from the mouth and upper airways, as it is from the lungs with cigarette smoking.

Chemical Agents and Animal Testing

Industrial agents have always been prime suspects in different kinds of cancers. While human exposure to a wide variety of toxic substances—including metals, dyes, hydrocarbons, dust, and radioactive material—has been investigated, no differences were noted for pancreatic cancer rates specifically. However, workers in metal industries and in coal and gasoline plants may have a slightly increased risk; the correlation between exposure to such chemicals and pancreatic cancer in hamsters is certain. On the other hand, the same chemicals will not cause pancreatic cancer in other kinds of animals.

This seems to suggest that chemical exposure is not an important cause of pancreatic cancer. It is interesting that, as opposed to other kinds of cancer, cancer of the pancreas does not occur naturally in wild or domestic animals, as far as can be determined.

Preventive Measures

The rate of pancreatic cancer is slightly higher in the better-developed countries of the world, although the difference is small compared to other common cancers. Some researchers have wondered if the extra fiber eaten in less-developed countries could help protect against cancer of the pancreas. Though there is no evidence that dietary fiber is responsible, one can imagine how such a protective mechanism might work. The pancreas is responsible for producing the enzymes that break down fats, proteins, and carbohydrates, allowing them to be absorbed in the bloodstream; fiber is undigestible carbohydrates. When large amounts of fiber in the form of grain and lightly cooked or raw vegetables are eaten, certain pancreatic enzymes are not needed, and the pancreas is put somewhat at rest. On the other hand, a diet high in protein and fat forces the pancreas to produce more enzymes. When the pancreas is activated and "stressed," it may be more sensitive to whatever causes cancer.

DETECTION AND DIAGNOSIS

Although it is not especially helpful, the oldest test used for pancreas cancer is the upper gastrointestinal X-ray examination, commonly called an upper G.I. The barium dye is swallowed, outlining the stomach and the duodenum (the first twelve inches of small bowel after the stomach). Since the outlet of the stomach and most of the duodenum touch the pancreas, a large enough pancreatic cancer may produce a noticeable indentation in the duodenum. Needless to say, this test is unsuitable for early cancer detection.

Ultrasonography, a test using sound waves instead of X rays, is useful for detecting cancer in many parts of the body. It relies upon the difference in sound wave reflection between a cancer and its surrounding tissue. Sometimes the difference is small and the cancer cannot be detected; intestinal gas and excess fat may occasionally obstruct a distinct ultrasound image. However, cancers larger than 2 cm (the size of a nickel) can often be imaged. The ultrasound test is particularly good at distinguishing a cyst from a solid tumor. This is very helpful insofar as a simple cyst is never cancer. Another advantage of ultrasonography is that one can obtain multiplane images, rather than the simple vertical and horizontal images produced by the CT (computerized tomography) scan. Ultrasonography is less expensive, more versatile, and more mobile than the CT scan and, significantly, does not use X rays at all.

While computerized tomography gives an X-ray image in only one plane, it is less dependent on the skill of the ultrasonography operator, and while imaging the pancreas, it also yields high-quality images of the nearby liver, kidneys, and bones. In some patients, the physician can tell beforehand which examination is the more promising, but many patients undergo both tests.

The lower limit of cancer size detectable with the CT scan, as with ultrasonography, is about 2 cm. With the guidance of either ultrasonography or CT scan, it is possible to insert a thin needle through the skin of the front of the abdomen and into the tumor itself. Some cells can be aspirated, or withdrawn, into the syringe, and then processed onto a microscope slide. Even though the number of cells is a small fraction of what would be obtainable on biopsy during a surgical exploration, it is usually enough for a definite pathological diagnosis.

If a mass can be seen by either ultrasonography or CT scan, there is as much as an 80 percent chance that cells from the mass can be obtained for microscopic study. However, if the cells obtained are benign, the physician or technician never knows whether the mass was missed and the sample taken from nearby tissue. In this case, the needle aspiration is repeated or an operation is recommended for certainty. Of course, if malignant cells are found, the test has been a great help. The needle aspiration procedure is performed with the patient under local anesthesia and, most often, on an outpatient basis. At present, it is a specialized procedure available only in the larger centers.

In endoscopy, a long, flexible tube, through which the physician can see the actual lining of the stomach and duodenum, is inserted through the patient's mouth, down the esophagus, and into the stomach. The endoscope allows the physician to inspect the duodenum, which touches the pancreas for most of its length. By examining the duodenum, and in particular the portion of the duodenum into which the main pancreas duct enters, the doctor can investigate for cancer of the pancreas. Biopsies can even be performed where the duct empties into the intestine. Though the biopsy size is small, about a sixteenth of an inch, it is enough to detect the cancer if present at that site. Unfortunately, only the end of the duct, which empties into the intestine, can be directly visualized.

Sometimes juice from the pancreatic duct can be drawn into the endoscope to allow microscopic examination for any shed malignant cells. In addition, it is possible for the entire pancreas duct system to be outlined with dye and made visible upon X ray by using an extension of the scope to inject dye into the duct itself. Although helpful in some respects, this is usually not an exact enough procedure for determining the existence of pancreatic cancer.

Summary of Diagnostic Tests

Several patients have asked me whether the availability of numerous tests for the detection of pancreatic cancer means that no one of them is regularly better than the other. Unfortunately, that is precisely the situation. As in all cancers, the best help is early detection. If one's vague abdominal discomfort lasts for more than a few weeks and a cause cannot be found, special tests should be recommended including ultrasonography or possibly a CT scan, depending upon which is more available and/or better perfected at a given testing center. If any mass appears, it should be biopsied, either with a needle under ultrasonography or CT scan, or through surgery.

Because pancreatic cancer is a highly lethal disease and because procedures to control it can be very punishing to the body, I believe that every diagnosis of pancreatic cancer should be confirmed by tissue specimen. One of the most striking features of this cancer is the low percentage of cases that are confirmed by biopsy. In fact, it is probably the lowest percentage of any cancer site in the body. A study conducted several years ago reported that only about half of the patients diagnosed to have cancer of the pancreas while alive actually had the disease, as proven at autopsy. The other half were found to have either cancers arising at other sites or nonmalignant diseases. This is due, in part, to the position of the pancreas in the back of the abdomen and its resultant inaccessibility, a fact which may also account for the late discovery of pancreatic cancer. Thanks to the recent and useful technique described above, a biopsy can be accomplished under local anesthesia with a needle of the size used for drawing blood. The few hundred cells the radiologist withdraws is often enough for an accurate diagnosis.

TREATMENT

Surgery

Two surgical approaches are currently employed for treatment of cancer of the pancreas: partial and total pancreas removal—and both have similar complication rates. The partial pancreas removal, called the Whipple procedure after the surgeon who first described it, involves removing the right side, or head, of the pancreas, where most cancers begin, and the nearby lymph nodes. Also, because the pancreas and duodenum are supplied by the same artery, the duodenum must be included in the surgically removed specimen, otherwise it would die from lack of blood supply. Since the bile duct connecting the liver into the intestine runs through the head of the pancreas, that duct is also removed with the specimen. The reconstruction of the remaining parts involves sewing the stomach, the bile duct, and the duct of the remaining pancreas back into the rest of the intestine at three places.

Follow-ups of patients undergoing the Whipple operation show that 5 to 15 percent do not survive the surgery or the immediate postoperative course. This mortality rate reflects the dimensions of the operation, one of the most extensive performed in abdominal surgery. Moreover, older patients with pancreatic cancer are often poorly nourished because of the cancer as well as other significant diseases. With a skilled and experienced surgeon, careful patient selection, and modern postoperative care, a pancreas removal can be performed at specialized centers with a lower mortality rate.

A particularly hazardous part of this procedure is the joining of the remaining pancreas duct to the intestine. In the days following the Whipple operation, this joining leaks in a certain percentage of patients. The strong digestive enzymes of the pancreas can then seep through the rest of the abdomen and cause the breakdown of other joinings or of the abdominal incision. Infection and occasionally hemorrhage, secondary to infection, can also complicate the postoperative course.

Removing the whole pancreas avoids the problem of pancreas duct leak. In addition, the complete removal avoids the problem of unrecognized cancer cells in the remaining pancreas. For these reasons, total pancreas removal has been generally advocated. One consequence of pancreas removal is the severe diabetes that follows. However, one or two kinds of insulin taken twice a day can rectify the situation. Enzymes (protein, fat, and carbohydrate digesting substances) produced by the pancreas can be replaced through various pills. Even with removal of only part of the pancreas, it is often necessary for the patient to take pancreas enzyme pills. A total pancreas removal has complications and mortality rates similar to a partial.

Even if the patient cannot be cured, surgery may be needed because the cancer mass may block the stomach outlet or the bile duct connecting the liver to the intestine. In either case, a segment of intestine can be joined to the area below the blockage, allowing the food or bile to detour and bypass the obstruction internally with no skin exit. More recently, it has become possible to drain the bile duct and relieve the jaundice by inserting a tube one-eighth of an inch or so in size through the blockage, without surgery. This placement, accomplished through the skin near the ribs, is done under X-ray control by highly specialized radiologists. It is appealing because the patient is not subjected to a major operation and lengthy recovery period when cure is not possible.

Radiation

Standard X-ray treatment, with cobalt or similar machine, is usually given slowly over eight to ten weeks instead of surgery or as supplemental treatment after surgery. Unfortunately, this procedure involves risks to the liver and kidneys, structures in the path of the X ray directed at the pancreas. Both organs are sensitive to high X-ray doses.

Intraoperative X-ray treatment, a technique involving the use of an external X-ray machine in the operating room, is available at eight to ten centers in the United States. During the surgery, important organs are either moved out of the way of the beam or covered by a sterile lead shield. Since the administration of a single high X-ray dose has not routinely increased survivals, research is under way to evaluate the combination of both a single intraoperative X-ray dose and the standard postoperative external X-ray treatment.

Implanting the cancer with radioactive isotope seeds has been tried at various cancer centers. The radioactive elements provide high-dose, short-distance charges that irradiate little more than the area actually around the seeds. Unfortunately, there are many complications, usually secondary to pancreas enzyme leak. Experimentation also includes the use of other high-energy beams, similar to X rays or gamma rays, but composed of neutrons, protons, and other particles. These specialized energy machines are available only at a few locations in the United States. So far, there is no data to suggest that they will produce better survival rates than standard X-ray equipment.

Chemotherapy

There are no particularly effective drugs for pancreatic cancer, as there are for breast and ovarian cancer. The two most commonly used drugs are 5-FU/fluorouracil or doxorubicin hydrochloride (Adriamycin). Recently, mitomycin (Mutamycin) and Streptozotocin have been used to treat this cancer, but they do not appear to be more effective. Only 10 to 30 percent of pancreas cancer patients receiving these drugs will show improvement.

Stomach or Gastric Cancer

T hough many people use the term to refer to the area between the chest and groin, the stomach is technically the food reservoir that connects the esophagus (swallowing tube) with the beginning of the small intestine (duodenum). The shape is that of the letter *J* or perhaps a Spanish wine flask with a longest dimension of twelve inches. It is flat when empty and can accommodate about three pints following a meal. The layers of muscle in the stomach squeeze and churn food, breaking it up mechanically and mixing it with digestive secretions. The glands of the stomach's lining produce hydrochloric acid, mucus, and enzymes to start the digestive process.

More than 95 percent of all stomach cancers arise from the lining, which is glandular; these cancers are called adenocarcinomas, or adenocancers ("adeno" means gland). Most cancers are located close to the lower outlet of the stomach, producing symptoms of stomach blockage as the cancer grows. As much as 10 percent of cancers diffusely involve the entire stomach.

About 25,000 people in the United States, two-thirds of them men, developed cancer of the stomach in 1984. The disease is rare in either sex before the age of forty and reaches a peak incidence between sixty and eighty years.

In 1930, when accurate statistics were first kept, stomach cancer was the leading cause of cancer death in the United States. Since then,

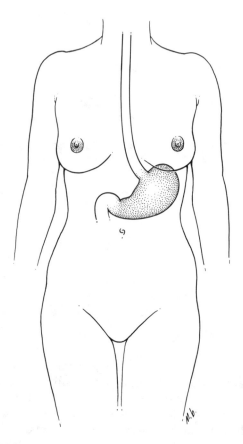

Shaded area indicates stomach

the rate of stomach cancer has declined dramatically in the United States, so that it now ranks eighth in frequency of occurrence and ninth in cause of death. Between 1930 and 1975, there was a 74 percent drop in the rate of stomach cancer among men and an 86 percent decrease among women. In Japan, however, stomach cancer still results in more deaths than all other cancers combined.

The overall cure rate for stomach cancer has remained constant over the past five decades, with 12 to 14 percent of those diagnosed surviving five years. (After pancreas and lung cancer, stomach cancer has the poorest cure rate of any common cancer.) If the cancer is treated before it spreads, the cure rate is 40 percent. But if at the time of diagnosis it has spread even to the nearby lymph nodes, only 15 percent survive five years. If the disease has spread to other organs—the liver being the most common—only 1 percent or less survive five years. Unfortunately, almost half the patients are diagnosed at this late stage.

SYMPTOMS OF STOMACH CANCER

- Ache or sensation of fullness, tightness, or discomfort in the upper abdomen.
- Sensation of fullness after a small meal.
- Sensation of food remaining in stomach for a long period.
- Blood in stool, usually noted as a black bowel movement.
- Rarely: nausea, vomiting, belching.

SYMPTOMS

The symptoms of stomach cancer often include some kind of stomachache, usually in the form of indigestion. Because such symptoms are familiar to everyone, they are usually not taken seriously, either by the patient or, on occasion, by the doctor. The symptoms may include fullness, tightness, or discomfort in the upper abdomen; nausea; heartburn; belching; loss of appetite; or, more specifically, the sensation of having had a large meal after eating only a little. Vomiting, weight loss, and anemia from unsuspected bleeding are sometimes later symptoms. If the cancer is located high in the stomach, tending to obstruct the esophagus, there may be difficulty swallowing, with food sticking at the affected point. Occasionally, blood found in the stool will lead to the diagnosis of stomach cancer even before the patient has any symptoms; these patients usually have the least advanced cases.

Stomach cancer symptoms are frequently confused with certain common conditions, the most frequent being stomach or duodenal ulcer, although hiatus hernia and irritable bowel can also display symptoms similar to those of stomach cancer. The symptoms of stomach cancer, in particular, can imitate those of duodenal or peptic ulcer, which occur at some time in about 10 percent of Americans. Both advanced stomach cancer and severe duodenal ulcer disease can cause blockage or perforation of the stomach, as well as blood in the bowel movement. While the pain of stomach cancer tends to occur immediately after meals, that of peptic ulcer tends to occur when the stomach is empty. In both cases, however, the pain may be improved with antacids. Unfortunately, over-the-counter and even prescription pills and liquids are taken so commonly that many stomach cancer patients mistakenly rely on them for several weeks before having diagnostic tests. It is probably wise to delay no longer than two weeks with self-medication before seeking a physician for a definite diagnosis. Certainly, if further tests show that the problem causing the symptoms is one of the benign and common conditions, several weeks of such medication is usually advised. However, should the tests reveal stomach cancer, several valuable weeks will not have been lost before beginning the correct treatment.

WHO IS AT RISK?

Immigrants from high-risk to low-risk countries experience a significant decrease in the rate of stomach cancer from one generation to the next as dietary practices adapt to those of the host country. This suggests that the malignancy has environmental, rather than genetic, causes.

Geographical Factors

The rate of stomach cancer is ten times lower in the United States than in Japan, where it causes about half of all cancer deaths, with no significant decline in recent decades. High rates are also present in such widely divergent countries as Iceland, China, Chile, and Colombia. Even among the close Scandinavian countries, Iceland and Finland have twice the rate of Norway and Denmark.

By moving to California, first-generation Japanese immigrants decrease their rate of stomach cancer as compared to those Japanese still living in Japan, although the rate is higher than that of the Californian white population. The second and third generation of Japanese immigrants—who tend to eat a more typically American diet—have a stomach cancer rate similar to that of native Americans. Dietary practices of migrant groups tend to adapt to those of the host country, as do customs and culture in general, over the succeeding generations.

Stomach Ulcers and Inflammation

Duodenal ulcers, the common peptic ulcers that affect 10 percent of Americans, are not associated with stomach cancers. Most authorities believe that ulcers of the stomach itself, which are less common than duodenal ulcer disease, are likewise unassociated with stomach cancer. Furthermore, most researchers have concluded that stomach ulcers do not become malignant, although a stomach cancer from its beginning can look similar to a stomach ulcer.

Previous surgery on the stomach may cause a predisposition to stomach cancer. In most instances of stomach cancer after stomach surgery, the patients had had part of their stomachs removed for duodenal ulcer disease more than fifteen years previously. In addition, most had had a reconstruction of the gastrointestinal tract that allowed bile to enter the stomach remnant, causing inflammation. It is more probable that the long-standing inflammation caused by the specific reconstruction, rather than the surgery itself, predisposes to stomach cancer.

Genetic Factors

The familial or genetic predisposition to stomach cancer has been studied with several different approaches. Examination of the rate of stomach cancer in identical, versus fraternal, twins suggests that there is no particular risk for closely related people. On the other hand, family members of a stomach cancer patient have about twice the risk of this disease, probably more for dietary, than for genetic, reasons.

Stomach cancer is associated with a lower socioeconomic status, whether the data are based on residential district, occupation, income class, or census tract information. Various confirming studies in Norway, Connecticut, Iceland, Hawaii, and Japan, seem to attest to the universality of the fact. Why poorer people should have a higher incidence of stomach cancer is unknown.

Diet

More than fifty reliable studies have been conducted around the world exploring the local dietary differences between stomach cancer patients and persons without the disease. Though the various studies have usually found different diets between the two groups, there is no single food common to stomach cancer patients. For example, in Japan, stomach cancer patients had eaten more dried/salted fish and pickled vegetables than the general population; in Norway, smoked fish; in Minnesota, bacon, fried foods, and cooked fat; and in England, flour and cooked cereal grains. The most consistent finding in all these studies is the significant preventive role of fresh fruits and vegetables.

Overall, the diet studies suggest that a high intake of processed grains and foods chemically altered—whether by salting, smoking, or pickling—may contribute to the development of stomach cancer. What these various foods have in common is not clear, although some contain nitrates or their derivatives, which are suspect materials. For example, foods preserved by salting contain far higher nitrate and nitrite levels than do similar foods preserved by refrigeration. Nitrates are commonly found in cured meats, as well as in cheeses and drinking water. When combined with normal mouth and throat bacteria, they can be converted to nitrites. These can be further converted to nitrosamines, from the addition of amines in fish products, processed grains, tea, and so on. Nitrosamine itself is found in minute amounts in bacon, sausage, smoked fish, and mushrooms. Experimental evidence in rodents suggests that nitrosamines, nitroso-ureas, and related compounds are a possible cause of human stomach cancer. In parts of Chile, Colombia, and England, a higher incidence of stomach cancer is found in those areas with a higher level of nitrate in the soil or water than in the surrounding areas. In one study, communities with a high incidence of stomach cancer in an otherwise low-risk area have been found to use nitrate-rich wells as sources of water.

The theory that stomach cancer is caused by chemically preserved food is compatible with the documented decline of this disease in the United States. Refrigeration started to become commonplace in the 1930s and 1940s. Before that time, meats, and foods in general, were preserved by smoking, salting, pickling, and drying—i.e., with the addition of possible cancer-causing agents. The thirties and forties also saw refinement in produce shipping and marketing, and fresh fruits and vegetables became more widely available. Citrus fruits and vegetables such as lettuce are high in vitamin C, which inhibits the formation of both nitrosamines and nitroso-ureas. This inhibition by vitamin C occurs both in the test tube as well as in experimental animals. In addition, some modern chemical additives, such as butylated hydroxytoluene (BHT), which are commonly added to bread, cereals, and other flour products as preservatives, tend to inhibit formation of these cancer-causing agents. The association of stomach cancer with a lower socioeconomic class may be due to nothing more than the greater relative expense of fresh fruits, vegetables, meat, and fish.

Other Risk Factors

Studies relating smoking and/or alcohol to the risk of stomach cancer are equivocal. Radiation also appears to have little or no effect on stomach cancer, except at the high levels to which few people are exposed. On the other hand, pernicious anemia, a disease characterized by thinning of the stomach lining, raises the risk of stomach cancer 500 percent. The lining is unable to produce a substance called "intrinsic factor," the presence of which is absolutely necessary for absorption of vitamin B_{12} from food. Why this disease should predispose to stomach cancer is as yet unknown.

Preventive Measures

Studies to date suggest that avoiding or decreasing the intake of foods altered by smoking, salting, or pickling or any other chemical processing may be helpful in preventing stomach cancer. On the other hand, greater use of fresh fruits and vegetables and other foods rich in vitamin C should be useful in blocking the formation of carcinogens. Since vitamin C tends to disappear with cooking and prolonged storage, the emphasis should be on "fresh."

DIAGNOSIS

Since the stomach is an abdominal organ, it is not easily evaluated by physical exam. Indeed, a stomach cancer would have to be large, and the person thin, before it might be felt.

Another difficulty in diagnosis is that stomach cancers imitate ulcers not only by producing similar symptoms but also by appearing as ulcers, whether viewed indirectly by X rays or directly by endoscopy. The older and more available diagnostic test is an upper gastrointestinal (UGI) series or X ray, but a small cancer may be missed or may appear to be a simple ulcer with this test. Therefore, UGI endoscopy with direct viewing of the lining and biopsy of any abnormality is a more reliable test.

X Rays

A UGI series is usually performed after a patient has fasted from eight to twelve hours. In the radiology department, the patient will drink several ounces of barium dye, a flavored chalky fluid, that will outline the contours of the esophagus and stomach. The radiologist may constantly view the whole process through fluoroscopy, which is a motion picture representation. Then permanent X-ray films are taken at various intervals in different positions—back, front, side—for later review. The procedure is painless and requires about two hours. Since barium tends to cause constipation, bowel movements will probably be irregular for the next few days.

To expand the normally collapsed stomach and allow the barium to thinly coat the stomach lining, the radiologist may introduce air into the stomach, usually in the form of effervescent tablets. This is called the double-contrast exam and is used more frequently in Japan, where many more stomach cancers occur.

Upper GI Endoscopy

In this procedure, a lighted, flexible tube less than one inch in diameter is passed into the stomach or duodenum through the mouth. The lining of the upper gastrointestinal tract can be seen and biopsies can be taken through the telescopic tube. (Endoscopy with rigid tube is performed with the patient under general anesthesia.) As with the upper GI series, fasting for about twelve hours is required to permit clear viewing of the tissue.

A local anesthetic gargle is applied to the mouth and throat to cancel the gag reflex; in addition, a short-acting sedative is given intravenously. A small mouthpiece is then placed between the teeth, and the doctor guides the tube down the patient's throat. The passage is aided by the patient's swallowing. During the exam, the patient feels unable to swallow, as the anesthetic liquid tends to make the patient's tongue and throat feel swollen. The exam is performed while the patient is lying on the left side (drooling saliva is wiped away with tissues). There is no real pain, though occasionally the patient may experience a cramp, if the duodenum, as well as the stomach, is examined. Since air is introduced into the stomach, it may feel full, although not uncomfortably so. Viewing the stomach may take thirty to forty-five minutes. Possible, though rare, complications include perforation (less than 1 in 1,000 times), bleeding at a biopsy site, and regurgitation and inhalation of stomach contents.

After the endoscopy, a patient may have a sore throat, which can be helped by lozenges. No intake of food or fluid is allowed until the effects of the IV sedation and the local throat anesthetic have worn off—usually within three to four hours. Otherwise, the patient could choke on the food or fluid. At this point the patient will be allowed to leave the outpatient area of the hospital, where this exam is usually performed.

Biopsy

Often a tiny biopsy, involving a sample of about one-eighth inch, obtained by UGI endoscopy, will reveal malignant cells on microscopic analysis. Sometimes the abnormality may look cancerous, but multiple biopsies will reveal only the inflammation that surrounds many stomach cancers. In these instances, surgery may be indicated. Sometimes the abnormality will appear to be a benign gastric ulcer, and multiple biopsies will *not* reveal any malignant cells. Then it is usually safe for the patient to undergo some six weeks of treatment for gastric ulcer and have a repeat UGI endoscopy to assure that the ulcer has healed and the stomach lining has returned to normal. However, in perhaps 10 percent of cases, both the visual appearance of the ulcer and the normal cells found on biopsy are misleading, and the abnormality is truly a cancer. Therefore, it is usually recommended that any stomach ulcer that does not heal completely within several weeks be treated by surgery for removal of that part of the stomach. Note that the above applies only to stomach ulcers, which must be followed closely. Duodenal ulcers are regularly treated by medications for years or even decades, because there is virtually no fear of cancer from ulcers of this site.

Early Detection

Because of the high incidence of the cancer in Japan, screening to detect cancers before they cause symptoms has been most highly developed there. The Japanese have detected early cases in mass surveys through the use of UGI series and a camera attached to the endoscope. They appear to have accomplished their ultimate aim of lowering the death rate from stomach cancer, even though they have not lowered its frequency. For example, the percentage of stomach cancer cases confined to the stomach lining was 3 percent in the mid-fifties and rose to 34 percent, due to the mass screening, in the mid-sixties. And because the large percentage of these were early cases, the overall survival rate from stomach cancers of those screened was 63 percent. When compared to 12 percent, the overall survival rate in the United States, one can see that screening and early detection do make a difference. However, since this malignancy is not common in the United States, and screening techniques are complicated and expensive, mass screening is not cost-effective in this country and has not been used.

TREATMENT

Surgery

Removal of part or all of the stomach with the draining lymph nodes is the only method known to cure stomach cancer. If the cancer has attached itself to the spleen and part of the colon and the patient appears curable, they too are removed. But stomach cancer is commonly at an advanced state at the time of diagnosis, so somewhat less than half of patients will undergo stomach removal. The usual location of stomach cancers is near the outlet, and partial or complete stomach blockage often results. Therefore, even if a patient cannot be cured—for example, because of spread to the liver—the surgeon still strives to remove the affected portion of the stomach to prevent any subsequent blockage.

The operation is a major one, involving an upper abdominal incision and three hours or more of surgery. In the case of a partial stomach removal, the remaining stomach is sewn to the small intestine. If the whole stomach is removed, the esophagus (swallowing tube) is sewn to the small intestine. The patient will require ten to fourteen days or more of postoperative hospital care. There is a complication rate of about 5 percent, the most common being infection, which would prolong the hospital course by several days. Two months after surgery the patient will have returned to all normal activities. Stomach cancer surgery does not usually require a skin or surface connection with the bowel, as is the case in a colostomy with rectal cancer surgery. Infrequently, a temporary tube may be sewn into the stomach, which exits just beneath the left rib cage. More frequently, a tube is placed through the nose to drain the stomach for the first postoperative days. It can be painlessly removed in a matter of seconds when no longer needed.

Fortunately, a person can live a normal life with only part (or even none) of the stomach, though diet is usually different after such surgery. Since the stomach itself is smaller, or even nonexistent, large meals cannot be eaten, and indeed only half the usual amount of food may give the same feeling of fullness. This fact usually necessitates four to six smaller meals per day. However, after several months, the remaining stomach will stretch and this aftereffect will lessen. Since the mechanism controlling the passage of the food contents from the stomach into the intestine is also removed in the operation, food that is not thoroughly digested may enter the small intestine, causing intestinal cramps and occasional diarrhea. At times, a person may even suffer from low blood sugar and consequent dizziness. The troublesome foods—usually liquid, sugary ones, such as milkshakes—and the other factors quickly become known to the patient and can be avoided. Slow eating and a diet of easily digestible foods are recommended.

Radiation

Stomach cancer is not particularly sensitive to X-ray therapy. The tissues around the stomach—such as the liver, spinal cord, etc.—are damaged by the high doses needed to destroy stomach cancer. These facts have largely limited the role of radiation to two goals: as a relief for pain (which often occurs with moderate shrinking of the cancer), and as an experimental aid to surgery in an attempt to produce better cure rates.

Chemotherapy

Combinations of 5-FU (Fluorouracil), doxorubicin hydrochloride (Adriamycin), and mitomycin (Mutamycin) have often been utilized. Chemotherapy has been somewhat more successful in stomach cancer (more patients respond) than in other gastrointestinal cancers. There are the usual side effects of chemotherapy with these combinations, including hairlessness, disease of white blood cells and platelets, nausea and vomiting, and mouth and throat sores. In addition, Adriamycin may damage the heart after accumulated doses.

Colorectal Cancer

While the most frequently occurring cancers are breast cancer in women and lung cancer in men, the most common cancer overall in men and women of the United States is that of the colon and rectum. There were an estimated 130,000 cases in 1984; about one in every twenty people born in the United States develops colorectal cancer. Colorectal cancer occurs equally among men and women, and its incidence increases with age. Although its 50 percent cure rate is better than that of many other cancers, it still accounts for 15 percent of all cancer deaths. It is the third most common cause of cancer death in women aged thirty-five to fifty-four and the most common cause of cancer death in those aged seventy-five and over, surpassing even breast cancer.

The large intestine, or bowel, the last part of the tubular gastrointestinal tract, is composed of the colon and rectum; it is called large because its average diameter is two inches, as compared to that of the small bowel, which is one inch in diameter. The small bowel empties its liquid waste contents into the colon at the lower right side of the abdomen. After traveling through an average of five feet of colon—and becoming more solid in the process—the waste material is deposited into the rectum in the lower midpelvis. The rectum, a tube seven inches long and three inches wide, ends at the anus, the skin and muscle opening between the buttocks. The various parts of the

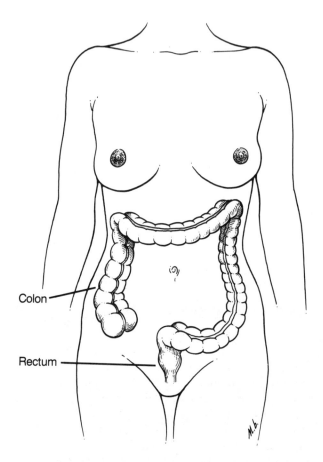

The colon and rectum

colon—cecum, ascending, transverse, descending, and sigmoid—are named to designate either their location or their shape. They are very similar to one another in function.

The colon removes much of the water and some of the last remaining nutrients from the liquid digested material it has received from the small bowel. The rectum stores the waste until it is expelled in defecation.

The innermost part of the muscular tube of the colon and the rectum is lined by a single layer of glandular cells, which absorbs water and secretes mucus to lubricate the passage of stool. It is in these cells that large-bowel cancers originate. They are therefore called adenocarcinomas or adenocancers.

SYMPTOMS OF COLORECTAL CANCER

- Blood from the rectum.
- Blood in the bowel movement.
- Changes: size of stool, frequency of movement, sense of incomplete evacuation, difficulty in passing stool.

SYMPTOMS

A change in bowel habits is one of the most important signs of colon and rectal cancers. These changes may include size of stool, difficulty in passing stool, cramps, frequency of movement (whether tending toward diarrhea or constipation), need for more (or fewer) laxatives than usual, or sense of incomplete evacuation. Any visible blood passed with, or mixed in, the stool, or blood from the rectum at other times, *must* be evaluated; it is a mistake to assume that one or two episodes of bleeding can be safely ignored. Bleeding from a cancer is often intermittent, especially in the early stages. And ignoring the bleeding episode (until it returns in several weeks) means that time for early detection will have been lost. Unfortunately, patients and even physicians often attribute bleeding to hemorrhoids—which the patient may indeed have—and waste valuable time on various hemorrhoid-related treatment. Sometimes blood in the bowel movement will have chemically changed so as to make the stool appear jet black. In such cases, slow blood loss with bowel movements will eventually result in a low red blood cell count, or anemia, and the patient will feel weak and easily fatigued. Later symptoms of colorectal cancer may include the presence of abdominal pain, bloating, or a mass in the abdomen. While some of these symptoms are more likely to be caused by colitis or polyps than by cancer, all of them should be promptly reported to one's physician.

WHO IS AT RISK?

Polyps

Polyps are merely growths of various sizes originating from the cells lining the colon. When large enough, they may bleed. More than half of all Americans will have at least one polyp in their lifetime; most patients never even know that they have a small polyp or two. This kind of polyp—whether it occurs singly or as one of several—is different from those due to familial polyp disease, in which hundreds of polyps are present at a given time. (See discussion on this genetic disease below.) Though common polyps are usually benign, the risk of their containing malignant cells increases with their size. However, even small, benign-appearing polyps can harbor malignant cells, which is why removal of all known polyps is recommended.

Large polyps and certain specific types of polyps are more prone to malignancy. However, it is not certain that the routine colorectal cancer—composed totally of malignant cells—originates in polyps. Whether polyps lead to cancer, or whether polyps and cancer are two separate diseases, is the cause of much debate. (Perhaps the most convincing evidence is found in animal experiments, where it has been demonstrated that polyps lead to cancer in the presence of some carcinogens.) Accordingly, it is recommended that all polyps be removed, even though research has not proved that human colorectal cancer originates from them. In a twenty-five-year study at the University of Minnesota, on 18,000 individuals, researchers performed annual sigmoidoscopy (examination of the sigmoid colon) with removal of any polyps. This program resulted in 85 percent less colorectal cancer over the twenty-five years than was predicted for the group. The study supports the suggestion that routine removal of polyps decreases subsequent development of cancer.

Polyps are more easily removed than one might think. There is usually no need for surgery. In fact, so seldom is surgery required that I would advise that the patient seek a second opinion when an abdominal operation for polyp removal is recommended. With use of one or another instrument (proctoscope, sigmoidoscope, colonoscope), any polyp can usually be lifted and detached at its base. The polyp is then microscopically analyzed to check for malignant cells. Curiously, the process of polyp removal cannot be felt, owing to the lack of nerves governing sensation. There is some discomfort caused by the presence of the scope in the anus and by the small amounts of air pumped into the colon, which gives a "gassy" sensation. For a colonoscopy (which requires the longest scope) and sometimes for the others, a mild drug, such as Valium, is given during the procedure. The most likely complication is bleeding at the site of the detachment; this, however, is rare. In the rare case where malignant cells are found upon microscopic examination, a subsequent abdominal operation is advisable for removal of that part of the colon.

Familial Polyp Disease

There are several inherited diseases, occurring in one in 5,000 to 10,000 people, which cause numerous premalignant colon polyps. In some of the inherited polyp diseases, colorectal cancer eventually occurs in every affected person. Under such circumstances, preventive removal of the colon and rectum in young adulthood is strongly recommended. As will be discussed below, all of the colon and most of the rectum may be removed, with the pathway for the bowel movement left unchanged. Removal of the entire rectum results in the bowel movement's exiting into a bag on the abdomen. Even though it is safer to remove the entire colon and rectum, some patients with inherited polyp diseases choose to have only the colon and some of the rectum removed. The small bowel is then connected directly to the remaining rectum. Without the colon and its water-absorbing ability, frequent diarrhea occurs until the body adjusts—usually within several weeks or months. The patient may then have two to three loose bowel movements a day, but no diarrhea. Although the patient's remaining rectum is still cancer-prone, early detection is possible; since the rectum is a short tube, a doctor can easily examine it with a gloved finger every three to four months. A doctor can also use a scope to visualize the rectal lining on a regular basis. Both scope and finger exam can be done in the office. Polyps can be detached and examined, and cancers can be discovered when very small. (An easy and thorough colon exam is not possible because the colon is not within reach of the finger.)

Colitis

In general, "spastic colon," or colitis, has no effect on the risk of colon cancer. However, two specific kinds of colitis—ulcerative and regional enteritis (also called Crohn's disease)—do increase the risk. The former increases it significantly; the latter, only slightly. The risk of cancer with ulcerative colitis increases with three factors: (1) the extent of rectum and colon involved, (2) the length of time the disease has been present, and (3) the severity or frequency of episodes. If an individual has had fairly active disease in both the colon and rectum for twenty-five years or more, the risk of developing colorectal cancer in the patient's lifetime is 40 percent. With a high enough risk factor, a preventive total colon and rectum removal may be recommended.

Does It Run in Families?

There is some evidence of a familial tendency in patients with colorectal cancer. The tendency probably depends upon multiple factors and perhaps more upon similar diets within families than upon genetics. There is some evidence that patients who develop colorectal cancer before the age of forty are more likely to have a familial predisposition than those developing it after forty. The risk among close relatives of patients with colorectal cancer is probably about two to three times that expected in the population at large. Thus, because the lifetime probability of any person's developing colorectal cancer is about 5 percent, its presence in a close relative (parents, siblings, and children) may double the probability.

Diet

With respect to colorectal cancer, comparison of the populations of Japan and the United States is most interesting. Japan has a high rate of industrialization, resulting in much pollution, and the Japanese ability to manufacture and export numerous goods has produced a high standard of living—comparable to that of the United States. However, the rate of colon cancer in the United States is four to five times higher than that in Japan.

The Chinese and other Asian people also have a low rate of colon and rectum cancer. Therefore, one might conclude that Asians are genetically less prone to colorectal cancer than are Westerners. However, that the differences are not genetic is clear from studies of migrant persons, whose cancer rate gradually changes in the new country. Observations of Japanese immigrants to California have shown that the colon cancer rate gradually increased over two generations to nearly equal that of the local white population. Clearly, factors other than genetics are at work.

One is diet. There are significant differences in the average diets of Asians and Americans. In the United States, about 40 percent of total calories are derived from fat, mostly saturated, and largely from dairy and other animal products. In contrast, the Japanese derive only 10 to 20 percent of their caloric intake from fat, of which a large amount is unsaturated. The daily average total fat intake is 152 g in the United States and 46 g in Japan. The daily cholesterol intake in the two countries averages 304 mg in Japan and 556 mg in the United States. In moving from a low- to a high-incidence country, the Japanese migrants developed more colorectal cancer than the relatives they left behind—though less than the native Americans. This may have occurred because the migrants adhered to the diet of their native land to a great extent. However, as their children's diet began to resemble the diet typical in the new country, the incidence of colorectal cancer increased accordingly. (The genetic makeup of the offspring remained the same throughout as it had been in Japan, because of continuing marriage within the immigrant group.)

If the consumption of meat creates the risk, vegetarians ought to have a lower incidence of colorectal cancer, even if they live where the disease is common. Studies have shown that Seventh-Day Adventists, most of whom are vegetarians, have about half the colorectal cancer as the American population at large. Other studies have attached less importance to meat as a cause of colon cancer. For instance, the Mormons, who eat meat, were also found to have a lower risk of colon cancer than the general population. However, they also eat a great deal of vegetables, most of which are homegrown and unprocessed. Given the considerable fiber intake, their diet can hardly be considered "typically American."

One investigator, who studied certain strong-tasting and unpopular vegetables, such as brussels sprouts, cabbage, turnips, cauliflower, and broccoli, theorized that large amounts of vegetables might be protective. He found that these vegetables induced a certain small-bowel enzyme activity in experimental animals. When these enzymes were added to the diet of experimental animals, the number of tumors caused by a particular carcinogen decreased. A Norwegian study suggested similar results in humans; its results showed that the rate of colon cancer was 25 percent smaller in people who ate large amounts of vegetables than in the general population. A study from the Roswell Park Cancer Institute in Buffalo, New York, yielded similar findings. Also intriguing is evidence from Denmark and Finland that suggests the protective role of cereal fiber. The incidence of large-bowel cancer among the Danes, as among Americans, is high; it is four times greater than that of the neighboring Finns. But while the fat and meat intake of both countries is approximately the same, the Finns consume nearly twice the amount of fiber, mainly in the form of whole rye bread. As a result, the Finns have greater and more frequent elimination than do the Danes. Accordingly, the rate of transit of digested material seems to correlate with a reduced risk of colon and rectum cancer.

PREVENTIVE MEASURES

A low-fiber diet appears characteristic of most countries with a high colorectal cancer rate, while high-fiber diets are prevalent in most countries with a low rate. Dennis Burkitt, a well-known advocate of the fiber theory, believes that a low-fiber diet may not be the factor responsible for colorectal cancer, but, rather, that the presence of high fiber protects against colorectal cancer regardless of its cause. In fact, according to his analysis, large-bowel cancer is one of a number of gastrointestinal diseases characteristic of modern Western culture, against which fiber-rich diets may afford some protection. Other bowel diseases against which dietary fiber has been found helpful or protective include appendicitis, diverticulitis, and hemorrhoids.

Diets rich in carbohydrates are almost always fiber-rich. In the United States, we often associate cakes and breads with carbohydrates. These foods, however, are usually highly processed and thus offer little fiber. The rest of the world's "carbohydrates" are whole grains as well as vegetables and fruits. The fact that Seventh-Day Adventists (vegetarians) and Mormons (with a large intake of cereal fiber and home-ground whole meal flour) have low rates, though they live in a country with a high rate overall, tends to validate the fiber theory.

How does fiber work to effect this protection? Fiber increases bowel movement bulk, which, in turn, may dilute possible cancer-causing agents. For example, fiber dilutes bile acids that find their way into the digestive tract from the liver. Certain bacteria found in large numbers in the colons of meat eaters chemically degrade bile acids into secondary bile acids. While not cancer-causing agents in themselves, secondary bile acids are thought to be "promoters"—that is, though they do not cause colon cancer in animals, they do increase the cancer rate when a known cancer-causing chemical is introduced experimentally.

The increased amount of stool caused by the additional fiber results in a faster transit time through the bowel. This presumably shortens the duration of contact between the cancer-causing agent—whatever it may be—and the cells lining the colon. Furthermore, some kinds of fiber, such as wheat bran, increase the acidity of the bowel movement. This may have an effect in decreasing the risk of colon and rectal cancer. Fiber may further protect by absorbing the presumed cancer-causing substances, thereby preventing their digestion and entry into the bloodstream. In the final analysis, however, it is not yet known how, or even if, fiber protects against colorectal cancer.

DETECTION AND DIAGNOSIS

Digital, or Finger, Exam

In terms of the number of lives it has saved by early detection, the single most important test for colorectal cancer is the finger examination of the rectum; of the approximately five feet of large bowel, the six-inch rectum is the most prone to malignancy. The examination is simply what its name implies: using the index finger, the doctor examines all the rectum within reach for any growths. The test is quick, highly accurate, and requires no special equipment or training on the part of the doctor, as do barium enemas or the various scope procedures. The finger exam is as important as stool blood analysis, with which it is usually combined, and should be part of every pelvic, as well as of any routine physical, exam. Considering the frequency of colorectal cancer overall and the frequency of the rectum as a particular site, it makes no sense to refuse a finger exam while obtaining other tests, such as a Pap smear or EKG.

Test for Blood in the Stool

After a digital rectal exam, the easiest and least expensive test, with an average cost of less than $5, is that performed on stool samples. This test can reveal small amounts of blood—even as little as one or two drops—invisibly mixed in the stool. Most cancers and even large polyps will bleed into the bowel movement. Although the amount of blood lost may be small, it is relatively constant in each stool, so that random samples usually reveal it. In fact, the test is so sensitive that patients are advised to avoid red meat before and during the stool sample collection. In addition, one should avoid vitamin C preparations and a few foods whose natural chemical contents may interfere with the test. A high-roughage or high-fiber diet with added raw fruit and lightly cooked vegetables is recommended. The extra indigestible roughage should irritate any possible growth in the large bowel, stimulating any previously unknown bleeding and making it more easily detected on the test. Peanuts, popcorn, and bran cereal also produce the same result.

The test has become so convenient and private that no one should have serious objections to doing it at home once a year. After following the simple dietary instructions for two days, one merely gathers a thin smear of the passed stool with a wooden stick and applies it to the inside of a cardboard container. Another sample is taken from another area of the stool. The whole process is repeated from the next two bowel movements in the following days, resulting in six stool specimens. The cardboard containers, which resemble matchbooks, are mailed back to the physician or lab. A chemical developing agent reacts predictably with any blood. Of course, the test can and should also be done on stool that the physician obtains on finger exam. The great advantage of a six-specimen stool test performed annually is that it makes it possible to find very small cancers—months and possibly years before they would produce any symptoms. The disadvantage is its nonspecificity. Blood demonstrated by this test can be caused by any number of factors, and additional tests are always necessary to reveal the actual source.

In one study of 900 apparently healthy individuals, the six-specimen test revealed blood in 5 percent. Of these, one-fifth had a colon cancer that had not yet caused symptoms; three-fifths had polyps or diverticulitis or some other nonmalignant cause; and the remaining fifth revealed no source even after numerous tests. (This might have resulted from failure to follow the diet carefully.) Of the patients who had colon cancer with no symptoms, almost all were cured.

Blood in the bowel movement is due to colorectal cancer about 10 percent of the time. It can also be the result of many other factors, including ulcer disease, nosebleeding, and eating rare meat. Moreover, benign growths in the form of polyps more commonly cause blood in the stool than do malignant growths or cancers.

X Rays and Scopes

Beyond digital examination and stool specimen tests, malignant and benign growths can also be detected by two general means: X ray and scopes. In the former, dye is introduced into the gastrointestinal tract to outline it for visualization on X ray. In the latter, a lighted, transparent tube, or scope, is passed into the gastrointestinal tract. The scopes for the rectum and colon can be rigid or flexible.

Barium Enema

This test is used to evaluate the function and anatomy of the colon and rectum. A typical functional problem that might necessitate a barium enema would be the rapid movement of the bowel resulting in diarrhea; among the causes are spastic colon, ulcerative colitis, or any kind of inflammation. An anatomic problem might be the suspicion of an enlarging growth that partly blocks the colon.

A patient prepares for this test by "cleaning out" the whole colon and rectum. Usually this involves taking only liquids on the preceding day, and fasting for twelve to sixteen hours before the test to keep the amount of stool at a minimum. In addition, on the day preceding the test, the patient takes strong laxatives and will usually have an enema. The patient can usually self-administer this enema, which comes in a prepackaged container with an insertable nozzle. This program should eliminate virtually all bowel contents that might interfere with the X-ray imaging.

The procedure for barium enema is as follows: on arrival, the patient changes into a hospital gown and lies on an X-ray table. A small rubber tube, thinner than a pencil, is passed into the rectum. While the patient lies flat, the doctor takes X rays at regular intervals as the barium dye gently flows in by gravity. Barium, which appears white or colorless, is not irritating, and the whole procedure feels no different than any other enema. When the barium has outlined the entire colon, the radiologist will ask the patient to turn to one side or the other to allow better visualization of a particular area. The patient is then allowed to expel the barium contents and to return for one more picture. In all, some five or six permanent films are taken. Some of the information is obtained by simple observation of the enema dye flow without the taking of a permanent X ray.

Sometimes a thin barium solution and moderate amounts of air are injected for the special visualization of small polyps. This is called an air-contrast barium enema.

Scopes

Proctoscope, sigmoidoscope, and colonoscope are names referring to the area that the scope can reach and examine. "Procto" refers to rectum. The proctoscope is about six to eight inches in length, the sigmoidoscope from twelve to fifteen inches, and the colonoscope more than thirty-six inches. The first is rigid, the second rigid or flexible, and the third is always flexible. Through these lighted tubes it is possible to examine every square inch of the rectum and colon and to remove polyps. Usually, the bowel will be prepared as if for a barium enema. However, less preparation is needed for proctoscopy than sigmoidoscopy, and less for sigmoidoscopy than for colonoscopy.

Not surprisingly, the expense involved and the training required for this equipment increase with the amount of bowel examined. In the late 1970s, the American Cancer Society dropped its recommendation that persons over the age of forty without symptoms have an annual sigmoidoscopy. The Society now recommends, instead, that examination be done on a three- to five-year basis on persons over fifty. Annual examination is appropriate for persons with high-risk factors and, of course, should be performed on any patient with symptoms.

The twelve-inch scope can find only 30 to 40 percent of cancers; the others will be beyond its reach. In various institutions, the highest number of cancers found was 1.5 per 1,000 patients without symptoms. However, 1 out of every 1,000 sigmoidoscopies will result in a complication. The colonoscope, by examining the large bowel, can find any colorectal cancer. However, this test is rather uncomfortable, can take thirty minutes to several hours, and requires both a specialist and the use of sophisticated equipment. Accordingly, the procedure is used only on patients with high-risk factors or specific symptoms.

TREATMENT

Surgery

Doctors almost always recommend that patients with colorectal cancer undergo surgical removal of the bowel segment containing the cancer—even if the cancer has spread and is incurable. If the bowel involved is not removed, continued growth of the cancer will usually cause a blockage of the bowels—or, occasionally, perforation or hemorrhage—necessitating a dangerous emergency operation.

The purpose of curative surgery is (1) to remove the cancer mass with enough large intestine to ensure removal of any microscopic spread in the intestinal wall and (2) to remove the draining lymph channels and regional lymph nodes. In most cases, if the cancer is on the right side of the colon, the entire right half of the colon is taken. If it is on the left side, most of the left side is removed. As surprising as it may seem, even if only a small part of the colon remains, there will be little or no change in bowel function. If the cancer is located in the rectum, the entire rectum is usually removed. A permanent colostomy, as explained below, results. None of these surgical procedures affects subsequent fertility and pregnancy.

The patient usually enters the hospital three or four days before the proposed surgery. Oral laxatives, enemas, antibiotic medication, and low-residue or liquid diets are prescribed. The surgical procedure requires ten to fourteen days in the hospital. Complications, such as infection, may extend the period.

The scar for a colon or rectal cancer is relatively long and usually vertical, from the top to the bottom of the abdomen. The incision allows for visibility of all the important abdominal organs. It is not possible to make a horizontal and more cosmetic scar close to the pubic hair, as is done for many gynecologic operations. If the rectum is removed, there will also be a scar around the former site of the rectum/anus.

Colostomy

The colostomy involves surgically attaching a part of the large bowel to the abdominal wall, allowing elimination into a bag. The actual visible colostomy is usually a circular protrusion of pink tissue above the skin, measuring about one inch in diameter. A colostomy can be permanent—as when the rectum is removed—or temporary to relieve a blockage and/or promote better healing, especially during urgent or emergency operations. It is usually located, especially if permanent, below the waist and near the hip. One must wait several weeks before a temporary colostomy is repaired, allowing for resumption of the normal bowel movement pathway. The closure of a temporary colostomy through an abdominal incision is a major operation in itself.

A rectal cancer usually necessitates removal of the total rectum, and a permanent colostomy results. If most of the colon remains, waste material will be generally solid, as would be the case under normal circumstances prior to surgery. Accordingly, the colostomy can be "trained" to function only once a day, usually with a self-administered morning enema. For the rest of the day, the colostomy is covered by a large dressing. A colostomy (without a bag) should not interfere with wearing any kind of clothing, even clinging knits. Certainly one can swim with no problem.

Ileostomy

If both the colon and rectum are removed, waste material exits through the small bowel. Though many refer to it as such, this is not really a colostomy, but rather an ileostomy, named after the last part of the small bowel (the ileum). Because the colon, with its water-removing and storage capability, is removed, waste material—about a quart of greenish liquid—forms throughout the day. An ileostomy cannot be trained, and a bag must be worn constantly. Moreover, the care of the surrounding skin and the bag appliance is more important. Since a bag is worn constantly, loose clothing may be more desirable.

Some patients are candidates for an operation to form a pouch of natural tissue inside the abdomen, allowing them to avoid wearing an ileostomy bag. The pouch can hold only four to six hours' worth of ileostomy contents. The patient must routinely evacuate the pouch with a small tube inserted through a tiny skin opening into the pouch. This system requires no external device or bag, and any kind of clothing, including bathing suits, can be worn. However, the Kock's pouch—named after the surgeon who popularized it—is still a new procedure with a reasonably high complication rate.

Special Treatments for Rectal Cancer

Since complete removal of the rectum results in a colostomy, other kinds of operations have been attempted. If the cancer is in the upper or midrectum and is not very large, it may be possible to save the lower rectum—the part most important for controlling the bowel movement. However, the chance of cancer's recurring in the lower rectum is higher, and it is not yet known whether the ultimate cure rate will be compromised.

If the cancer is truly small, superficial, and growing outward instead of into the bowel wall, it may be possible to remove the cancer by a cautery cutting device. Cautery does not remove bowel around the cancer or the lymph nodes. For this reason, it is an inadequate curative operation, but rather a halfway measure for those who cannot physically withstand a larger operation or those who refuse a colostomy.

Radiation

Because of the tendency of rectal cancer to recur in the original area, X-ray therapy to the pelvis is frequently recommended. The temporary side effects include cramps and diarrhea, as well as burning and stinging of the skin around the anus and the genitals. The X-ray treatment may be given three or four weeks following removal of the rectum.

Many specialists prescribe preoperative radiation. Though this can make the following operation more difficult, it seems to decrease the chance of cancer's returning to the pelvis. In preoperative radiation therapy, the blood and oxygen supply of the cancer remain intact, theoretically making the X-ray therapy more effective.

X-ray treatment is uncommon in areas of the colon beyond the pelvis, since there is only a small tendency for colon cancers to recur locally. However, both pelvic colon cancers and other colon cancers can spread through the bloodstream, an occurrence not prevented by X-ray therapy.

Chemotherapy

If the lymph nodes of the surgical specimen contain cancer cells (but the cancer has not spread to distant parts of the body), the cure rate is less than 50 percent. As of yet, no known postoperative treatment improves these statistics. This situation differs from breast cancer, in which drug treatment of women with cancerous lymph nodes appears to increase the cure rate by preventing, or at least delaying, recurrence of cancer.

The most common sites of distant spread are the liver, lungs, and abdomen. If the cancer has recurred, various drugs, such as 5-FU/fluorouracil alone or combined with mitomycin (Mutamycin) or with one of the nitroso-ureas (for example, BCNU or carmustine) are used. Besides lowering the blood cell counts and causing temporary nausea and diarrhea (which is common to these drugs), 5-FU may also cause mouth sores.

Kidney Cancer

The kidneys are bean-shaped structures roughly six inches in length that are located behind the organs of the abdomen, just beneath the back muscles. As illustrated, they lie high under the ribs, just below the diaphragm. The kidneys act as filters, removing waste products from the blood, while returning all other substances to the circulating blood supply. The central portion of the organ is hollow and collects the urine from the kidney filtration units. Urine leaves the kidneys by exiting the hollow portion (called the collecting system) and passing down the ureters, tubular structures about eighteen inches long, which connect the kidneys to the bladder.

Cancers of the kidney comprise less than 2 percent of all malignancies in adults. About 1 in 700 to 800 people can be expected to develop kidney cancer. The age of peak incidence, as in most genitourinary cancers, is fifty to sixty years, with three men developing kidney cancer to every one woman. In 1984, an estimated 18,000 cases were diagnosed in the United States. About 50 percent of kidney cancers are localized to the kidney and have spread neither to the lymph nodes nor to any distant organ at the time of diagnosis. In these patients, the five-year survival, or cure, rate is 70 percent. The overall cure rate—including all patients with kidney cancer—was 42 percent a decade ago, and is slightly higher at present.

The cell of origin for 80 to 90 percent of kidney, or renal, cancer

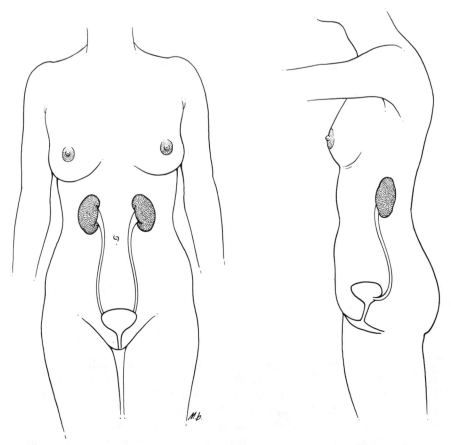

Front and side views of kidneys. Shaded areas indicate kidneys.

is that composing the renal filtration system. It is sometimes called clear cell cancer because of the transparent appearance of its cells under microscopy. In the rare instance when cancer originates in the kidney's collecting system, the malignancy behaves like a cancer of the bladder.

SYMPTOMS OF KIDNEY CANCER

- Blood in the urine—often intermittent.
- Pain radiating down flank or side.
- Vague ache or pain in the kidney area.

SYMPTOMS

Blood in the urine—either visible to the naked eye or diagnosed on laboratory analysis—is found in over half of all patients with kidney cancer. The blood is usually present during the entire act of urination rather than at the beginning and/or middle, as is more common with bladder cancer. There are usually weeks or months in which the urine clears up temporarily and then becomes bloody again. Radiating pain down the side occurs in about a third of the cases. The pain may be caused by blood clots passing from the kidney to the bladder and may be the same as that caused by kidney stones. However, the pain can also be vague and remain confined to the kidney area. Swelling on the side of the body with the kidney cancer may accompany the pain. Other associated abnormalities include fever (7 percent), weight loss (28 percent), and anemia (21 percent).

Sometimes the cancer is found by an IVP (intravenous pyelogram) before it produces symptoms (see the section on bladder cancer for a description of this test). A patient may undergo an IVP for other reasons, such as kidney stones, and be diagnosed for cancer. Cancers found this early are curable almost twice as often as routine kidney cancers that have already produced symptoms.

WHO IS AT RISK?

The cause of kidney cancer is unknown, but because of the greater frequency in men, male hormones have been suspected. In both laboratory animals and humans, radiation is believed to cause kidney cancer. There is a slight but definite increase of kidney cancer caused by cigarette, pipe, or cigar smoking, and by tobacco chewing. One study found that men under age fifty who smoked one pack of cigarettes per day had eight times the rate of nonsmokers. Other studies have not shown as marked a difference between tobacco users and nonusers.

On a worldwide basis, the rate of kidney cancer is higher in northern Europe and North America than in Africa, Asia, and South America. Moreover, the fact that kidney cancer occurs more frequently in men who tend to be occupationally exposed to industrial chemicals has spurred the search for causative agents, though none is currently known. There is no tendency for kidney cancer to run in families, although a few rare chromosomal diseases, such as von Hippel-Lindau disease, do predispose to kidney cancer. Because there is no known cause, there are no definite preventive measures that can be taken. From its association with tobacco, proven more in some studies than in others, it would certainly seem prudent to stop using all forms of tobacco.

DIAGNOSIS

Tests for kidney cancer include urinalysis, IVP, and tomograms. Urinalysis is the microscopic study of cells in the urine that have been collected by a centrifuge. The procedure allows even blood cells too sparse to be seen with the naked eye to be visualized with the microscope. Blood in the urine can result from a stone and/or infection at any point in the urinary tract. Upon discovery of blood in the urine, an IVP is performed, and, for increased precision, a tomogram is usually done at the same time. The tomogram is an X-ray "slice" in which the levels above and below do not appear on the film.

Once a "spot" is seen on IVP, a CT scan or an ultrasound test is usually performed to determine whether the abnormality is fluid-filled (i.e., a cyst) or solid. Cysts are usually not malignant. Sometimes cyst drainage with a needle under CT scan or ultrasound visualization will make surgery unnecessary. Moreover, the CT scan often determines whether the cancer has invaded the organs surrounding the kidney and whether the lymph nodes, liver, or bone is involved. This is necessary for accurately staging the disease and choosing the appropriate treatment.

Because lungs, liver, and bone (in that order) are common sites of spread, a chest X ray, sometimes accompanied by liver and bone scans, may also be performed.

TREATMENT

Surgery

The treatment of kidney cancer is primarily surgical. If removal of the kidney is contemplated, a renal arteriogram (also called an angiogram) will probably be performed. In this hospital test, performed with the patient under local anesthesia, the renal artery is outlined by an injection of dye. The distribution of blood supply both in the kidney and the main vein draining the kidney is also made visible. For this procedure, a small catheter is inserted through the major artery at the groin and advanced up to the kidney artery. Understanding the blood supply and its involvement with the cancer is crucial to kidney removal.

Kidney removal is recommended for anybody with cancer localized to the kidney and lymph nodes (and not yet spread to the liver, lung, brain, or bones), since chemotherapy and radiation therapy are not especially effective and certainly cannot cure this disease. Total removal of the kidney along with the surrounding fat, lymph nodes, and the adrenal gland is usually performed through a horizontal incision at the back and side. A small group of patients with only one area of cancer spread outside the kidney may also undergo kidney removal, provided the growth in the single area is also removable. A small percentage of people with such limited spread may have long survivals or may even be cured.

Luckily, anyone can live normally with only one healthy kidney, as evidenced by the many people who have given up a kidney to a relative for transplant. It is probably wise for such people to avoid contact sports and dangerous physical pastimes in order to protect their remaining organ. Although very few women in childbearing years have developed kidney cancer, there should be no problem with successful pregnancy after the woman has completed treatment. Furthermore, one healthy adrenal gland is also sufficient. No hormone replacement or medicines are necessary.

Immunotherapy

If kidney cancer returns, it may not do so for ten years or more after the surgical treatment, suggesting that immunological mechanisms are important for keeping the cancer in check. A small group of patients (about 1 percent) who have a cancerous kidney removed will have spontaneous shrinking of the cancer in distant organs, giving further indication that immunological control may be significant. Coupled with the knowledge that renal cancer does not respond well to chemotherapy or X-ray therapy, these factors have prompted some investigators to try immunotherapy.

Unfortunately, passive immunotherapy (the giving of immune substances) with interferons and other agents has not proven very successful in treating renal cancer. Active immunotherapy (stimulating the individual's own immune system to produce such substances) in the form of tumor vaccines is now being attempted. One study shows a 25 percent improvement in five-year survival rates of patients who were treated with a tumor vaccine. In order to make a vaccine from an individual's cancer, however, the cancer must grow in the laboratory in tissue culture, and only half do so. The tumor cells are deactivated by certain agents. They are thus unable to reproduce within the person once the cells themselves, or subcomponents of the cells, are injected. A vaccine made from another person's kidney cancer may also be as effective as that made from one's own. At this early date, however, one cannot predict how useful immunotherapy will eventually be.

Other Treatments

Radiation therapy to the area from which the cancer has been removed is sometimes used as an additional treatment to destroy any microscopic deposits of cancer cells. Conventional chemotherapy may utilize such drugs as lomustine, or CCNU, and vincristine sulfate (Oncovin). Pain in a cancerous kidney that cannot be removed may be temporarily relieved by an arteriogram, which clots the kidney's blood supply. Rarely, a mild hormone called progesterone will temporarily shrink the cancer.

Bladder Cancer

T he bladder, located in the front of the lower abdomen, is the urine's reservoir. A circular organ in men, it is crescent-shaped in women with an indentation produced by the uterus. The bladder measures about an inch in diameter when collapsed; it expands to three to four inches in diameter when full, holding twelve to sixteen ounces of fluid. Although it is immediately adjacent to the uterus, the bladder is unrelated to sexual functions.

Urine, the liquid waste produced by filtration through the kidneys, passes through two thin tubes, or ureters, into the bladder. Eighty percent of bladder cancers are located where the ureters enter the organ, at the base of the bladder. Such cancers may obstruct the ureters, resulting in backup of urine, which can cause kidney failure. By virtue of its receiving, and extended storage of, concentrated waste products, the lining of the bladder is more exposed than other tissues to chemicals excreted in the urine. Whether situated at the base of the bladder or elsewhere, the vast majority of bladder cancers in this country and in all developed countries arise from the so-called transitional cells that line the bladder and much of the urinary tract. Only 6 to 10 percent of bladder cancers arise from the other cells present in the lining.

Thirty thousand new bladder cancers are diagnosed in the United States each year, resulting in about 10,000 deaths. Bladder cancer that

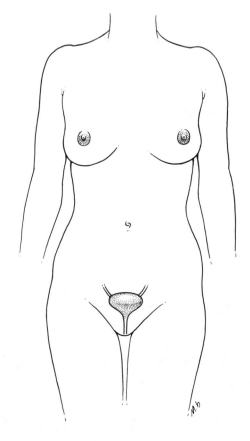

Shaded area indicates bladder

has not yet invaded the bladder muscle has a cure rate of over 80 percent. But those that have traversed the bladder wall and are present in the surrounding fat have cure rates of less than 25 percent. Of the 30,000 new cases, only about 7,000 occur in women. This lower incidence is also apparent in most other countries. In both sexes, incidence rises with age, and peaks in the sixth and seventh decades.

SYMPTOMS OF BLADDER CANCER

- Visible blood in urine.
- Invisible blood in urine revealed by urinalysis.
- Symptoms of cystitis: voiding frequent small amounts and urgent sensation to urinate.

SYMPTOMS

The presence of blood in the urine is the most common symptom in patients with bladder cancer; in one representative study, either visible or microscopically detectable blood was the first symptom in 85 percent of the patients. The study also noted that blood in the urine had been present for three to eight months before the patients sought medical attention. As with all cancers of the urinary tract, including kidney and bladder, the bleeding is usually intermittent. This means that it is essential that any bleeding, whether prolonged, or present in just one voiding, must be investigated. The study showed no relationship between the cancer and the amount of bleeding: some small cancers produce much blood.

Blood in the urine is not usually associated with pain. However, bladder cancer may cause bladder irritability—the frequent voiding of small amounts of urine, burning on urination, or the urgent sensation of having to urinate. These symptoms may result from the tumor's pressing upon the bladder wall. These same symptoms are often the result of the irritation and inflammation of the bladder—usually owing to infection and treatable with antibiotics—known as cystitis. Since cystitis is a hundredfold more common than bladder cancer, the physician is likely to turn to antibiotics before considering other diagnoses. However, if a patient has cystitis symptoms, but no infection is revealed by urine cultures, bladder cancer should be suspected. In fact, since cystitis may coexist with bladder cancer, patients may undergo a week of antibiotics to cure infection. Then, if any symptoms or bleeding in the urine persist, investigation for the possibility of bladder cancer should go forward.

Because the most common cancer site is the bladder base, near the urethra (the bladder's outlet), passing urine may seem hindered. A patient may experience hesitancy during voiding, an increased effort needed to void, and a decrease in the force of the urinary stream. Later symptoms may include low abdominal pain, weakness, and weight loss. Occasionally, the weakness and weight loss is due simply to the loss of considerable blood in the urine, which the patient has ignored.

WHO IS AT RISK?

Cigarette smoking definitely increases the chances of developing bladder cancer and probably doubles the risk. The higher incidence in men may result from the fact that traditionally so many more men than women have smoked; nonsmoking men and women have approximately equal rates of bladder cancer and lower rates than those of smokers. Researchers have estimated that a third of all new cases of bladder cancer are directly attributable to cigarettes. In fact, the increase in women smokers may be expected to produce a proportionate increase in the number of bladder cancers in women.

There is no predisposition to bladder cancer in one's genetic makeup. There is also no evidence for any "protective" foods, such as fiber in colorectal cancer.

Occupational Agents

Several industrial agents are known to be associated with bladder cancer. As early as 1895, an increased incidence of bladder cancer was noted in aniline dye factory workers. (Aniline is a simple substance that forms the basis for various colored dyes.) But when the aniline-related chemicals were first tested, they failed to cause bladder cancer in several kinds of animals, leading to the conclusion that these chemicals were not the cause. However, dogs and humans have enzymes that transform the aniline chemicals into cancer-causing agents, while other animals do not, and when dogs were exposed, bladder cancer resulted. The tests demonstrated the long latency period between exposure to the cancer-causing agent and the cancer's actual appearance: aniline dye workers develop bladder cancer after an average of sixteen years. Severe and prolonged exposure of industrial workers to an aniline by-product, beta naphthylamine, resulted in the development of bladder cancer in more than half the workers tested. Aniline compounds are absorbed through the skin, then eliminated through the urine. The cancer-causing agents could exert a cumulative effect through their daily storage in the bladder over several years.

Other chemicals suspected of causing bladder cancer are found in a variety of industries and include chemicals similar to aniline dye, including naphthylamine (encountered by rubber and cable workers), aromatic residues (common in the petroleum industry), and benzidine (to which medical personnel are exposed). Hairdressers, leather finishers, spray painters, and textile workers use similar chemicals, but appear to experience no increased rate of bladder cancer.

At the very least, occupationally exposed individuals should probably undergo regular bladder cancer screening examinations, such as urine cytology (the microscopic study of cells shed in the urine) as well as urinalysis (a simple test that will reveal red blood cells). The average age of individuals dying from bladder cancer caused by industrial agents is about fifteen years younger than patients with spontaneously occurring bladder cancers. Needless to say, any smoker in the aniline industry would be expected to have a particularly high risk of bladder cancer.

Artificial Sweeteners

As most people are aware, artificial sweeteners have been widely discussed in relation to bladder cancer. Early studies reported no increased risk in patients who regularly used saccharin or cyclamates (an artificial sweetener taken off the market several decades ago), but the number of patients analyzed in those studies may not have been large enough for detecting a small, increased risk of bladder cancer.

The link between cancer and artificial sweeteners rests largely on findings in animal studies. The use of animals in establishing the cancer-causing potential of artificial sweeteners has been criticized—unfairly—because the dose, as in similar studies, so greatly exceeds any human intake. However, the validity of the findings rests on the fact that cancer causation results from the inherent property of the chemical, independent of dosage and dosage duration. In other words, while a high enough dosage of *any* chemical may kill the test animal, only certain chemicals will cause cancer. Cancer-causing chemicals can be identified more quickly with high doses in small animals.

One recent study in humans has actually detected a slightly increased risk of bladder cancer among those who always use saccharin in place of sugar. As the widespread use of artificial sweeteners is still a relatively recent phenomenon, it is possible that the increased risk of bladder cancer may not become fully apparent for some years.

The fact that women are assumed to use saccharin so much more than men, and yet have a much lower rate of bladder cancer, may mean that the artificial sweetener has little, if any, influence on the development of this cancer.

DIAGNOSIS

Beyond the appearance of blood in the urine, testing for bladder cancer also involves bimanual examination. In this exam, the doctor places one hand on top of the abdomen near the pubic bone and one or two fingers of the other hand in the rectum or vagina. By compressing the bladder, the doctor can then evaluate any cancer large enough to be felt. However, since cancers must be quite large in order to be felt in this manner, bimanual examination does not help in early detection.

X-Ray Images

X-ray viewing is almost always performed first because it involves almost no discomfort or risk to the patient. However, in some instances, such as when the patient is allergic to dye, X rays may be deleted from the diagnostic test sequence.

X-ray viewing of the bladder, the next test, is possible in two ways: an IVP (intravenous pyelogram) and a cystogram. In the IVP, the dye comes "from above," since it is injected into the bloodstream, and is excreted by the kidneys into the urine. The IVP may show the bladder cancer itself or it may show blockage of a ureter that is caused by the bladder cancer. This visualization is not as accurate as that provided by a cystogram, a procedure wherein the dye is inserted "from below." Through a catheter temporarily placed in the urethra, the bladder is filled with approximately one cup of X-ray dye. No anesthesia is necessary. Many women have been catheterized, usually in relation to childbirth, and know that it is not painful. As the dye is withdrawn through the catheter, further films are made. While the normal bladder wall collapses evenly, a cancerous wall collapses irregularly.

Urine Cytology

Cytology—the study of individual cells—has been a significant tool in diagnosing some cases of cancer. In suspected cases of bladder cancer, for example, cells shed into the urine can be collected and microscopically examined. Because cancerous cells are less capable of adhering to one another than are healthy cells, the cancerous part of the bladder lining will shed its cells more readily than the healthy part, thus allowing detection. Unfortunately, such studies of urinated specimens cannot detect every cancer, so diagnosis of bladder cancer is not usually limited to so simple a test as urine cytology.

Cystoscopy

Cystoscopy can be performed under local anesthesia, but a short general anesthetic is more commonly used because of the discomfort involved. With either kind of anesthesia, the patient will remain in the hospital only several hours or a day. Cystoscopy and biopsy are the most important means of assessing bladder cancer for treatment. The cystoscope is a narrow, perhaps one-half inch in diameter, lighted telescopic tube that is inserted through the urethra, the point at which urine exits the body. Unlikely as it may seem, given the size of the urethra, instruments such as biopsy forceps can be manipulated and maneuvered through this tiny scope. This procedure is performed with the patient's legs in stirrups, as in a pelvic exam. Afterward there is only a small amount of discomfort, usually with stinging during the first few urinations.

Though cancer cells are abnormal by definition, there are degrees of abnormality. Those cancer cells that microscopically resemble normal cells more than most other cancer cells are called well differentiated. These cells grow neither as quickly nor as aggressively as those less resembling normal cells, called poorly differentiated. Biopsy will reveal the differentiation of the particular bladder cancer, which will be of use in planning treatment.

Staging

Many women are familiar with the term "staging" in cervical cancer. As in cervical cancer, the staging in bladder cancer involves determining the extent of the disease at the time of diagnosis. This determination, in turn, dictates the comprehensiveness of the treatment. Staging is also important for studying the results of different kinds of therapy, since a particular treatment may appear to cure more patients when they are diagnosed with less extensive disease. One commonly used staging system distinguishes progressive extension of the cancer into (1) the lining alone, (2) the supporting tissue beneath the lining, and (3) the actual muscle of the bladder or the fat outside the bladder. In addition, some staging systems take into account the resemblance of cancer cells to normal cells under the microscope. As noted previously, well-differentiated cancer cells (those more like normal cells) are associated with a slower-growing and less aggressive course. These cancers usually require less radical treatment. Conversely, the poorly differentiated cancers usually require more treatment.

TREATMENT

Low Stages

Treatment of low stage and superficial cancers can be performed without a surgical incision. This is accomplished by removing the malignant tissue through the cystoscope—the narrow, pencil-sized tube inserted through the urethra—that is used for biopsy and diagnosis. Since the pathologic exam of the biopsy requires a permanent section, the removal procedure is performed at a separate cystoscopy. With the patient under general anesthesia, the cancer is removed cystoscopically by fulguration—with electrical current. The bladder wall is left intact, demonstrating again that only superficial disease is amenable to this treatment. Because new tumors have been known to grow in the same vicinity in about a quarter of all these cases, patients will require cystoscopy every three or four months afterward. If no recurrences are found, intervals between exams will eventually be lengthened.

Occasionally, cancer-killing drugs are introduced through a catheter into the bladder. The procedure brings chemotherapy into direct contact with the bladder lining containing the cancerous growth. However, this is often not as effective as removal by cystoscope because the cancers recur. Administration of chemotherapy in this fashion is an experimental technique for those who refuse bladder removal, which is the safer procedure for superficial but widespread disease. Cobalt or external beam X-ray treatment also cause cancer shrinkage, though cancers tend to recur.

In patients whose superficial low-stage tumors recur quickly, especially if they involve an increasing area, the preferred treatment is to remove the bladder and construct a stoma, or external exit, allowing for the urine's collection in a bag at one's side. Although this may seem drastic for low-stage and superficial cancers, disease that continues to recur over the years is aggressive in its own way. When the disease recurs again and again, it may become high-grade at any time and prove fatal. Accordingly, after several recurrences of superficial disease, an extensive operation is usually recommended.

High Stages—Surgery

Treatment of deep or higher stage bladder cancer is more comprehensive from the outset. If the cancer extends into the bladder wall, even if the affected area is small, the best treatment is removal of the whole bladder, usually combined with radiation therapy. The portion of the vagina that contains the urethra, the outlet tube of the bladder, may also be removed. The clitoris will remain, but since some sexual nerve pathways are removed during the operation, sexual climax may be difficult afterward. The narrowed vagina may also make sexual intercourse difficult.

Given the difficulties of so extensive an operation, some patients have wondered why only the cancerous part of the bladder is not removed. For this to be possible, a cancer would have to be very small and situated precisely on the bladder "dome." Unfortunately, few cancers are so situated; some 80 percent are located at the bladder base. In the final analysis, only 3 to 5 percent of patients are suitable for partial bladder removal. This operation has fallen into disrepute, as physicians have tried to "stretch" the indications in attempts to spare patients the more extensive procedure. Indeed, rapid recurrence is the frequent result of a partial bladder removal when used nondiscriminately. Even if the cancer were small and in the correct location, a 1979 study showed that when the cancer cells were poorly differentiated, *all* patients suffered recurrence after partial bladder removal.

Radiation

Preoperative X-ray treatment is usually employed before bladder removal, since radiation reduces the size of the tumor and should prevent any cancer cells shed during surgery from growing. Preoperative X-ray treatment does, however, increase postoperative complications, since the effect of radiation is adverse to wound healing. The combined treatment results in three to five postoperative deaths in every hundred patients.

For patients who refuse bladder removal, even though the cancer has already invaded the bladder wall, X-ray treatment is offered; unfortunately, the cure rate is less than one-quarter of patients so treated. The X-ray treatment requires seven to ten weeks and can result in complications to the rectum as well as to the bladder. With the X-ray induced scarring, bladder capacity can be substantially reduced, resulting in urgency and frequency in urination. Such X rays will also cause ovarian failure and premature menopause.

Urinary Detour

The bladder is usually removed along with the adjacent lymph nodes. In the past, the problem of the urine's leaving the body was handled by sewing the ureters into the large bowel near the rectum, thus allowing patients to evacuate urine with their bowel movement in a diarrhealike mixture several times a day. Continence was thereby achieved and a bag was not necessary. However, severe complications, involving either ureter obstruction or infection from the mixture with stool, both of which might lead to kidney failure, often resulted. For these reasons, the method most widely used today for detouring the urine calls for joining the ureters to an isolated loop of bowel and bringing one end of the loop to the surface of the skin, where it is covered by a bag. The risks of obstruction and infection are minimized, since the loop remains unconnected with the rest of the bowel and prevents mixture with the stool. About half the time taken for this lengthy operation is spent in adapting a segment of small bowel for attachment to the ureters. The actual skin exit is called a stoma, the same term used for colostomies. The result requires a constant bag appliance, because urine is formed around the clock. Since urine is thin and watery and tends to leak, the technique of fitting the appliance with skin cement must be taught by a stoma therapist. Even though one must empty the bag every four hours or so, the bag appliance itself is left in place for five to seven days. One showers or bathes while wearing it. All kinds of colored and lacy bag coverups are now available. In addition, some patients use a short lacy top, like a teddy lingerie outfit, for sexual activity. The uterus and ovaries will be intact after surgical treatment, which would permit childbearing.

Chemotherapy

Standard chemotherapy, injected through the bloodstream, is not very effective against bladder cancer. While Cytoxan, Adriamycin, and cisplatin are most commonly used, it is clear that better drugs have yet to be developed for this particular cancer.

Brain Cancer

There are about 11,000 cases each year of cancers arising in the brain, but overall, they account for only 2 percent of all cancer deaths. Men have 1.4 times the number of brain cancers as women. About 85 percent of brain tumors arise in adults, peaking between the ages of fifty and sixty. Some kinds of brain tumors occur only in children, and brain tumors in general are the second cause of cancer death in children after leukemia.

The human brain weighs only twelve ounces at birth and about three pounds when fully developed. And yet, it can store more information than a library. It contains some 15 billion nerve units, which permit the processing and storing of information. The soft brain is encased and protected by the bony skull. At the base of the skull is the opening through which the spinal cord passes down the bony spinal, or vertebral, column.

The brain is composed of the cerebrum, cerebellum, and brain stem. The surface, or cortex, of the cerebrum is formed by the nerve cell bodies. Fibers from these bodies lead inward from the surface to form the inner part, or white matter. The fibers crisscross so that those entering the brain from the left side of the body cross over to the right side of the brain. Accordingly, the right half, or hemisphere, controls most of the left side of the body, while the left half controls the right side. The cerebrum is divided in half by a deep groove, with each half

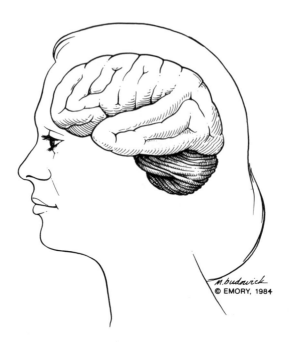

The brain

consisting of four lobes. The frontal lobe, adjacent to the forehead, contains nerves that affect emotional responses, attitudes, and thought processes. The parietal lobe, located in the midcentral area, contains nerves associated with sensation and motion. The temporal lobe is located adjacent to the temples and has to do with hearing. The part of the cerebrum farthest back is called the occipital lobe and is concerned mainly with visual perception. The cerebellum is located just below the occipital lobe, above the nape of the neck, and affects muscular coordination and equilibrium. The brain stem is the lowest part of the brain and becomes the spinal cord. The brain stem neurologically controls breathing, heart rate, blood pressure, and other functions that occur without conscious effort. The brain and spinal cord are covered by three layers of meninges (membranes), the outer part of which is a dense, fibrous layer. Between the two inner layers of meninges, the cerebrospinal fluid (CSF) circulates and acts as a shock absorber to cushion and support the brain and spinal cord within the bony skull and vertebral column.

The cell of origin in more than 50 percent of brain cancer cases is the nerve tissue itself, as in the tumor glioma ("glio" means glue, which the soft brain tumor resembles in appearance). The cell origin of approximately 15 percent is the meninges, as in a meningioma. Several rarer tissue sites constitute the remainder.

More tumors spread to the brain from their origins elsewhere than arise spontaneously from the brain itself. Although these are not true brain tumors, they frequently produce the same symptoms and are diagnosed by the same tests. All adults with brain tumors must be carefully evaluated because of the possibility of a tumor elsewhere. (When a child has a brain tumor, it invariably arises from the brain tissue and not from other organs.) The cancers that most frequently spread to the brain are those of the lung, breast, and kidney, as well as melanomas.

Unlike breast cancer, which is dangerous precisely because it spreads to life-supporting organs, brain tumors virtually never spread to other parts of the body. Brain cancer is particularly problematic for two reasons. First, within a given location it interferes with the neurologic function specific to that location. Second, its growth in the nonexpandable bony skull causes pressure on the entire brain.

SYMPTOMS OF BRAIN CANCER

- Headache—generalized and throbbing, worse in morning and sometimes associated with vomiting.
- Interference with any neurologic function: drowsiness, impaired speech, balance problems, limb weakness, seizures, loss of smell, lack of coordination, eye or facial muscle weakness, hearing loss, ringing in the ears, or personality changes.

SYMPTOMS

The symptoms of brain cancer may be caused by either generalized intracranial (within the skull) pressure or destruction of brain tissue at the tumor site. Headache is a common symptom of increased intracranial pressure and is usually generalized and throbbing. Characteristically, the headache awakens the patient in the early morning; in some patients, it also recurs intermittently throughout the day, often in paroxysms. Some patients have episodes of vomiting soon after they arise or at the height of the headache attack. Vomiting caused by brain cancer is usually not associated with nausea and may come suddenly, without warning. (Headache in young children should be considered an important symptom because children normally do not have headaches. In one study, headaches were present in 70 percent of children who were diagnosed as having brain tumors.) With the generalized pressure, the optic nerves are often also affected, but this rarely causes a detectable decrease in visual acuity. Occasionally, double vision may result from the increased pressure.

Any or all brain functions may be hindered or seriously impaired because of the destruction of a given area by the growing tumor. Diverse symptoms may result: drowsiness, impaired speech, balance problems, limb weakness, seizures (convulsions), loss of smell, changes in personality, lack of coordination, eye or facial muscle weakness, hearing loss, or ringing in the ears.

The typical migraine headache does *not* resemble one caused by a brain tumor. The migraine headache is usually preceded by nausea, but rarely by vomiting. It comes at any time of day and is usually localized to one portion of the head, or one side of the head. Likewise the twenty-four-hour-a-day tension headache is seldom caused by tumors or serious diseases. Infectious diseases resulting in brain abscesses are frequent causes of increased intracranial pressure and various neurologic deficits. Brain abscesses are usually associated with severe infections elsewhere. Other conditions that may cause either increased pressure and/or certain neurologic deficits are bleeding inside the brain (a form of stroke) or a subdural hematoma (clotted blood within the skull pressing on the brain, usually as the result of head injury).

WHO IS AT RISK?

Various rare chromosomal or genetic diseases predispose to brain cancer. These include von Recklinghausen's disease (neurofibromatosis), tuberous sclerosis, and von Hippel-Lindau disease. Except for these rare diseases, brain tumors do not tend to run in families. People who received head X-ray treatments as children several decades ago (to treat fungal disease of the scalp) have a slightly higher incidence of brain cancer. Aside from this, however, there are no data connecting irradiation with brain cancer. Most researchers agree that a past instance of head trauma—skull fracture or concussion, for example—does not increase the risk of brain cancer. At present, it is not believed that viruses cause human brain cancer, although particular viruses can cause such tumors in animals. Vinyl chloride, a chemical that was frequently used in plastics manufacturing, is linked with increased numbers of brain tumors, as well as with cancers of other sites.

DIAGNOSIS

A plain X ray of the head will show the bony skull. Only calcifications of the tumor will reveal the presence of a malignancy on plain X ray. CT (computerized tomography) scans are probably the most useful di-

agnostic test, although brain scans, arteriograms, and electroenceph-
alograms (EEG) may sometimes be helpful. If a brain tumor is
suspected, a CT scan may be the first and perhaps the only test prior
to surgery. However, an arteriogram is often needed before the operation, depending on the location and nature of the brain tumor, to
produce a "map" of the blood vessels. Because of its accuracy, if a CT
scan has been performed there is often no need for a brain scan. The
EEG is an ancillary test performed to investigate seizures.

CT Scan

A CT scan is a three-dimensional computerized analysis of multiple X-ray films of the skull and brain in successive layers. The variation in density of each tissue type allows for variable penetration of
the X-ray beam. An attached computer calculates the amount of X-ray
penetration of each tissue and displays the results in shades of gray.
The final result is a pictorial series of anatomic cross sections of the
brain and skull. Sometimes an X-ray dye is injected intravenously to
enhance the visualization of an abnormality. The normal brain tissue
is to some extent protected from the dye's entry by blood-borne substances. But abnormal brain tissue, caused by tumor or bleeding into
the brain, has enhanced dye uptake, which can be visualized well on
X-ray film.

In many instances, CT scans eliminate the need for more complicated procedures, such as an arteriogram (see below). There are no
complications associated with CT scanning other than an allergic reaction to the iodine dye (the same as used in intravenous pyelo-
grams). The amount of irradiation received in a CT scan is comparable
to that of three or four standard X rays of the head.

During the actual test, the patient lies on a table in a quiet, cool
room, which is necessary for the computer's function. The face is not
covered, but the patient's head fits inside a rubber cap—similar to the
bonnet on a hair dryer. Special pillows are placed alongside the patient's head to prevent small movements, since even those that accompany talking or sighing will ruin the picture. Usually, scanning is
first done without dye injection and is then repeated with the dye circulating. The entire procedure requires about an hour and can be performed on an outpatient basis.

Brain Scan

Since the recent development of the CT scan, some patients who
would have received brain scans in the past now receive only CT scans.
Brain scans are used mostly for patients who have spread of cancer
to the brain from sites in other organs. Brain scans are cheaper,
quicker, and more generally available than CT scans. In this test, the

brain is scanned after the intravenous injection of a minute amount of a radioactive isotope. The normal brain has a barrier that prevents substances in the blood from entering the brain tissue. However, in areas abnormal because of tumor or bleeding, the normal barrier is disrupted and isotopes tend to localize there. A Geiger counter recognizes this increase and displays it graphically.

This study has virtually no complications. There is no discomfort, except from the needle puncture for the injection of the isotope. Shortly after the injection, the patient lies on her back, side, and front while the Geiger counter measures the radioactivity, which leaves the body within twenty-four hours. There are no special precautions—whether one is an outpatient or an inpatient—because only trace amounts of the isotope are used.

Electroencephalography (EEG)

The EEG is a display of the electrical activity generated from the brain. It is very similar to an electrocardiogram (EKG), which records the electrical impulses of the heart. This study is invaluable in the investigation of seizures (epilepsy), but is not often performed when diagnosing a brain tumor unless seizures are the first sign.

Brain or Cerebral Arteriography

Arteriography—the injection of dye into the artery system, which will then outline the brain arteries—is a more complicated test than most, but is sometimes necessary before brain surgery. An artery, most often in the groin, is chosen as the puncture site for the insertion of a catheter. Although the skin site is numbed with an anesthetic, an artery puncture is significantly more painful than a puncture of a vein, the common site for any blood test. Guided by X rays, the catheter is passed up the arterial system and stops near the artery feeding the brain. This part of the procedure does not hurt. Indeed, there is no sensation from the movement of the catheter. When the dye is injected, however, the patient will feel a severe burning sensation in the head. Fortunately, this lasts only a few seconds. The catheter is then removed from its entrance site, and pressure is placed on the arterial area, which has a naturally greater tendency to bleed than do veins. The patient is then confined to bedrest for twelve to twenty-four hours with the leg flat—in the case of the groin—to allow complete sealing of the artery. Pulses beyond the arterial puncture site, for example, the ankle, are checked frequently to monitor possible complications, including closure of the artery.

The complications include possible bleeding and obstruction of the artery at the site of the arterial puncture. In rare instances, such a complication could require a repair operation on the artery. Another complication may be the dislodgment of a fatty plaque or clot in the brain artery, obstructing the blood supply and causing stroke. Although rare, both complications occur more frequently in patients with arteriosclerosis (hardening of the arteries), a condition common in older people.

TREATMENT

Surgery

The ideal treatment for most brain tumors is removal of the entire tumor, which often requires several hours of surgery. Some tumors grow with a capsule around them and can be completely "shelled" out. Other tumors extend into the normal brain tissue, like the roots of a tree, and the neurosurgeon must remove as much as possible without damaging any important normal tissue. Sometimes the roots grow back slowly and may require that the tumor be re-operated upon several times for removal over a period of years.

The operation itself is called a craniotomy, because the skull (cranium) must be opened. Preoperatively, the patient will be given steroids—to reduce brain pressure—and antiseizure medicine. A portion of the skull is removed and is replaced at the end of the operation to restore a normal head contour. The surgery is performed through this window, which is situated over the tumor. The skull heals as any bone fracture might and regains normal strength. The head must be shaved preoperatively, but when the hair grows back, even the skin scar is invisible. Many such procedures are performed with the operating microscope, which allows better visualization of the tiny, delicate structures.

After the operation, the patient may be quite sleepy and unresponsive for several days because of brain swelling and consequent intracranial pressure caused by the surgery. Swelling and bruising may also be seen in the soft tissues of the face. Because of the internal and external swelling, the patient is kept in a sitting position and not allowed flat for the first several hours. The main complication is oozing at the site of the tumor, with extra blood taking up space within the skull and putting pressure on the brain. Such complications may require immediate reoperation to relieve the pressure. After a craniotomy, the usual hospital stay is ten days to three weeks. Often the first few days are spent in the intensive care unit (ICU). The patient should be out of bed and able to take fluids in twenty-four to forty-eight hours. Seizures may occur as the result of any brain surgery, whether for tumor, injury, or any other reason. They are usually easily controlled by daily oral medications.

Radiation

X-ray treatment is used as the sole therapy when surgery is too risky—as when the patient is too fragile because of other health problems—or when the tumor is positioned where severe neurologic dysfunction will result from surgery to that area. Tumors located in the brain stem, for example, are routinely treated by X ray rather than surgery. X ray, especially when administered immediately after an operation (as for diagnosis), may produce signs and symptoms similar to those of the tumor. Nausea, drowsiness, and worsening of the original neurologic defect may result from brain swelling caused by the X-ray treatment. About a quarter of patients experience trouble thinking and other neurologic problems, which may develop immediately or within several weeks of X-ray therapy, because of the swelling. High doses of steroids are used to treat this problem. Irradiated parts of the skull usually experience permanent hair loss.

Chemotherapy

Chemotherapy for brain tumors is limited because of the blood-brain barrier, which usually prevents substances circulating in the body from reaching the actual brain tissue. A few drugs, such as BCNU, CCNU, and procarbazine hydrochloride (Matulane) are of a molecular structure that allows passage. After chemotherapy, the condition of about 10 percent of patients will become worse before it improves. The temporary deterioration is due to an increase in tumor size, swollen by the dead and dying cells. Therefore, worsening may indicate that chemotherapy has been effective.

Tumor Recurrence

Additional chemotherapy with different drug combinations may occasionally be effective, particularly when the tumor has developed resistance to the original drugs. Reoperation for a recurrent tumor is considered when the patient has done well for a prolonged period after the first operation. In one study of patients selected for reoperation, about 60 percent improved, and almost half of those remained improved for a year or more. If the tumor recurrence is in an area that has not yet received X ray, then that is a possibility. Although repeat irradiation in previously irradiated tissue is hazardous, it is occasionally performed.

Sarcoma (Cancer of the Bones and Soft Tissues)

S arcoma is a rare malignant tumor that originates from tissue connecting, surrounding, and supporting the various body organs. In this respect, its origin is fundamentally different from most cancers that arise from the lining of an organ (such as cancer of the bladder or gastrointestinal tract), from the duct system within an organ (such as cancer of the breast and pancreas), or from the functional cells within the organ itself (such as those of the thyroid or kidney). In fact, sarcoma is so different that the other cancers (comprising more than 80 percent of malignancies) are termed carcinomas in order to distinguish them from sarcomas.

The majority of sarcomas arise from the cells of the mesoderm, a loose network of cells first found in the embryo three weeks after fertilization. Because the mesoderm gives rise to many kinds of tissue, more than sixty different kinds of sarcoma have been identified. In addition to their common embryologic origin, sarcomas resemble each other in symptoms, microscopic appearance, and course of disease, thus remaining clearly distinct from other cancers. This type of cancer tends to occur equally in men and women. Because of similarities in behavior, tumors arising from Schwann cells (a class of cells that surround nerves but do *not* arise from mesoderm) are also included under the term sarcoma.

Sarcomas are roughly divided into those originating from the bone and those originating from soft (connective) tissue. About 1,900 cases of bone sarcoma occurred in the United States in 1984, mainly in the form of osteogenic ("osteo" means bone) sarcoma and Ewing's sarcoma, an even rarer form. Both subtypes of bone sarcoma occur mostly in children and teenagers. Chondrosarcoma ("chondro" means cartilage) and fibrosarcoma ("fibro" means fibrous) are considered bone sarcomas if they arise from that particular kind of bone tissue. Their greatest incidence is in the fourth, fifth, and sixth decade. Soft tissue sarcomas comprise many subtypes and are more widely distributed among all ages, with half occurring in patients between forty and sixty. In 1984 there were about 4,900 new cases of soft tissue sarcoma (with a resultant 2,400 deaths) in the United States.

Soft tissue sarcomas may arise from a variety of tissues: sarcoma originating from fibrous tissue is called fibrosarcoma; from fat, liposarcoma; from blood and lymph vessels, angiosarcoma and lymphoangiosarcoma, respectively; from smooth muscle, leiomyosarcoma; from striated muscle, rhabdomyosarcoma; from the lining of the joint, synovial sarcoma; from nerves, neurogenic sarcoma; and from cartilage, chondrosarcoma. Each of these has a benign counterpart: for example, fibroma from fibrous tissue; lipoma from fat; hemangioma from blood vessels, and so on. In most instances, benign tumors are not thought to become malignant; benign tumors remain benign, while malignant tumors are malignant from the beginning. The exception occurs in an inherited genetic disease, called von Recklinghausen's disease. In about 10 percent of these patients, neurofibrosarcomas originate from multiple benign neurofibromas.

More than half the body consists of soft tissue alone, regardless of body weight. Despite the large amount of bone and soft tissue from which sarcomas may arise, this kind of malignancy represents less than 1 percent of cancers in the United States. However, in spite of their rarity, sarcomas have generated much medical research because of their tendency to occur in young people: of those younger than fifteen years, sarcomas comprise 7 percent of all cancers. A generally poor cure rate, and the drastic surgical procedures, often including amputation, contribute to the interest in sarcomas.

Osteogenic sarcoma and Ewing's sarcoma tend to occur in the shafts of the longest bones, the thigh bone, or femur, being the most common site. The larger of the two calf bones, or tibia, and the upper arm bone, or humerus, are the next two most common sites. Soft tissue sarcomas occur throughout the body. Approximately half occur in the leg, with the vast majority in the thigh. Ten percent occur in the upper extremity. Approximately 15 percent occur in the retroperitoneum, the area behind the abdominal organs, a site with a particularly poor cure rate. The remainder of soft tissue sarcomas occur in the head, neck, and trunk.

Sarcomas Versus Other Cancers

After removal, sarcomas tend to recur at the original site with greater frequency than other cancers. For some sarcomas, the microscopic "roots" extend six inches or more beyond the obvious tumor. These roots can cause the malignancy to recur at the same site—and the cure rate to decrease—unless an extensive procedure is performed. Further, sarcomas tend to spread *not* through the lymphatic vessels and on to lymph nodes as do other cancers, but to the lungs first.

Although sarcomas can arise in many organs, they should not be confused with the so-called common cancer of the organ. For example, 95 percent of stomach cancers arise from the glandular lining and are therefore adenocarcinomas, or adenocancer. However, about 1 percent of stomach cancers arise from the smooth muscle just beneath the lining and are called leiomyosarcoma. The course of this disease is unlike that of the common stomach cancer, and the cure rate of leiomyosarcoma is much better. Other organs may give rise to sarcomas in the same way. As in other cancers, the size of the cancer and the degree of spread at the time of diagnosis determine treatment. The initial treatment for sarcoma tends to involve all three modalities—surgery, radiation, and chemotherapy—more often than with other cancers. Because of the rarity of sarcomas and the new and complicated treatment involved, patients should be treated at a cancer center by experienced physicians. To do otherwise would be to risk not obtaining the most recent and promising treatment.

SYMPTOMS OF SARCOMA

- Painless enlargement, usually in the limb, but also in the trunk, head, and neck.
- Occasionally: pain preceding awareness of the mass.
- Rarely: decrease in muscular strength or joint motion.

SYMPTOMS

Symptoms of sarcoma are variable and depend on the location of the affected bone or soft tissue. At first, the sensation of a mass or pain is subtle and intermittent, although the most frequent sign *is* the finding of a painless lump. On occasion, pain precedes awareness of the mass. The pain, if present, is first mild and fleeting, and then dull and aching (like a toothache), with localization to the area. Pain does not usually increase with activity, nor does it respond to rest, though increased pain at night, enough to keep the person awake, may be noted. Rarely will a patient first experience a decrease of muscular strength or joint motion. In only 5 to 10 percent of patients with bone sarcoma, the first sign is a fracture as the result of a minor injury.

Most patients are diagnosed with a relatively large lump, which has often developed over several months. Though some people may be able to remember an injury to the area, the injury merely calls attention to the presence of the sarcoma and has nothing to do with its cause. If the sarcoma is in the arm or leg, patients are likely to consider the problem as a "muscle pull," perhaps with bleeding into the muscle (hematoma). However, enlargements due to hematoma, torn muscles, or other muscle injury rarely last beyond three weeks, and those persisting longer should be evaluated for sarcoma.

WHO IS AT RISK?

Bone Sarcoma

Radiation is the only agent clearly associated with bone cancers, particularly osteogenic sarcoma, chondrosarcoma, and fibrosarcoma. Bone sarcomas occurred in 4 percent of women employed as radium watch dial painters before 1930; radium, used as dial paint because the radioactivity glowed in the dark, was swallowed when the women licked the paintbrushes to make fine tips. Once in the body, radium resides in the bones more than in other tissues. Six percent of patients treated with radium in the late 1940s for bone tuberculosis also developed osteogenic sarcoma. These cases appeared after a latency period of four to twenty-two years. However, of bone cancer patients, the fraction that had radiation exposure is small—less than 1 percent of all patients.

No chemicals have been proven to cause bone cancer in human beings, though some chemicals cause the corresponding malignancy in animals. Beryllium, a metal element, causes osteogenic sarcoma in rabbits, and vinyl chloride, used to produce plastic, causes it in rats.

Particularly in connection with osteogenic sarcoma, the role of infectious agents has been questioned by several laboratory observations. Viruses cause the malignancy in mice and chickens; extracts of human osteogenic sarcoma cause the disease in hamsters; questionable viruslike particles can be found in human tissue and in the tissue culture of osteogenic sarcoma.

There appears to be no increased risk to relatives of patients with bone cancer. There are, however, a few uncommon genetic or chromosomal diseases that generally cause maldevelopment of the skeleton and predispose to bone sarcoma. For example, Paget's disease, which causes thickening of the bone, particularly in the pelvis and skull, and affects mainly middle-aged and elderly people, also causes a twenty-fold increased risk of osteogenic sarcoma. However, with only 500 cases of osteogenic sarcoma per year in the United States, and most occurring in people between the ages of fifteen and nineteen, few patients have had Paget's disease as the predisposing cause. Paget's disease is slightly more common in the United Kingdom, as is sarcoma.

The common age for osteogenic sarcoma is fourteen in males and thirteen in females. It tends to occur during the adolescent growth spurt, which occurs approximately one year earlier in females. Some researchers believe that malignant tumors develop more rapidly in the growing bones that produce taller individuals; the most common site for osteogenic sarcoma is the femur, the longest bone in the body. In studies of dogs, the giant breeds develop osteogenic sarcoma more often than smaller breeds. Although the difference is much less dramatic in humans, children with bone cancers are taller than other children their age.

Soft Tissue Sarcoma

A small proportion of patients with soft tissue sarcomas have rare genetic diseases. The most common of these is neurofibromatosis, also known as von Recklinghausen's disease, which occurs in 1 out of every 2,500 live births; *The Elephant Man* is a story about an individual with a severe form of this disease. People with von Recklinghausen's disease have multiple lumps that are benign neurofibromas. However, in about 10 percent of these cases, one or more of these undergoes a malignant transformation to become a neurofibrosarcoma. As a general rule, the benign counterpart of a sarcoma—for example, lipoma for liposarcoma—never becomes malignant. Occasionally, though, the transformation of the benign counterpart to malignant can be caused by X-ray treatment—as with the X-ray therapy of hemangioma of several decades ago.

Kaposi's sarcoma, recently associated with Acquired Immune Deficiency Syndrome (AIDS), is thought to originate from either lymphatic or blood vessels. The disease is also more common in groups with suppressed immunity, whether the suppression is caused by drugs or other diseases. Apart from such groups, Kaposi's sarcoma is more common in African blacks, where it accounts for 5 to 12 percent of cancers in some countries. Although rare in Western Europe and the United States, it occurs mainly in men of Mediterranean and Jewish background.

As with bone sarcoma, there appears to be no increased risk for those related to patients with soft tissue sarcoma. Patients who have had one sarcoma do not seem at increased risk for development of another. Radiation plays little or no role in development of soft tissue sarcoma. Foreign bodies placed in soft tissue, such as breast augmentation and facial implants, do not predispose to an increased risk. Certain chemicals, such as inorganic arsenic (used in insecticides) and vinyl chloride (used in plastics manufacturing), may cause liver angiosarcoma, a rare disease numbering only a few dozen cases a year. Viruses have been identified in bird, mouse, rat, and cat sarcomas. As far as human research is concerned, there are particles seen in various human sarcomas that resemble those associated with viruses in animal sarcomas. However, such bits of information are suggestive at best and merely indicate further directions of research.

DIAGNOSIS

Biopsy is necessary to determine whether a tumor is a sarcoma or one of its benign counterparts. It is crucial to determine the type of sarcoma involved and its grade (the degree of abnormality when viewed microscopically). The grade is more important for planning treatment in sarcoma than in other cancers. All lumps in soft tissue or bone should be biopsied. Approximately 90 percent of sarcomas will recur if they are removed with no surrounding margin, so it is always wise to make the best attempt at treatment the first time.

On arms and legs, biopsy incisions should normally be placed vertically because of the direction of the blood supply, although a horizontal incision may at times be more cosmetic. A vertical incision allows for better healing if subsequent radical surgery is necessary. Also, it is best to keep the incision away from skin directly over the bone (e.g., the shin and ankle). Since these areas do not heal as well as those with fat and muscle beneath the skin, this factor may become important if surgery or X-ray treatment is later performed. Given the rarity of cancers of the soft tissue and bone, with the average pathologist seeing less than one a year, the microscopic slides should be reviewed at a cancer center by experienced pathologists.

If a biopsy reveals sarcoma, other tests are performed to check diligently for further spread of the disease and to determine precisely the involvement at the original site. Since virtually all sarcomas spread first to the lungs, a chest X ray followed by chest tomography and/or chest CT (computerized tomography) scan are necessary. (Tomography is an X-ray exam in which a sequence of films is taken, each representing a "slice" of the lung, usually a half inch apart. The slice clearly delineates the particular plane, and blurs out all other planes, making lung diagnosis more accurate than with conventional chest X rays.

The image of computerized tomography results from passing X rays through the patient's chest at a variety of angles. The variation in, and thickness of, each tissue allows for variable X-ray penetration. The varying penetration is given a numerical value called a coefficient, which is digitally computed to shades of gray. The final display appears as an actual photograph of the area sliced by the X ray.) Neither test has any complications, nor requires any injections, although X-ray dye is sometimes injected for CT scans of the chest to visualize the blood vessels.

It is of primary importance to determine whether the cancer is arising in the bone or whether it has spread from a malignancy originating in another organ. A bone sarcoma usually arises at one site, whereas cancer spread to the bone usually involves multiple sites. Although plain X rays of the entire skeleton will often determine this, a bone scan, which is a more sensitive test than plain X ray, is sometimes necessary. With this test, the entire skeleton is examined a few hours after the intravenous injection of a radioactive material. Normally this short-term isotope is distributed uniformly throughout the bones. An increased concentration is abnormal, and may represent a tumor, as well as arthritis or an injury.

In planning strategy before surgery and/or X-ray treatment, a number of tests are performed to evaluate the extent of involvement at the original site. These usually include plain X rays, CT scans of the area, and/or arteriography. The CT scan is usually done on both the normal and abnormal part (e.g., the right and left thighs) for the sake of comparison. The CT scan is so highly developed that it usually shows the exact extent of cancerous spread to the nearby muscles, as well as to the major artery/vein/nerve complexes. The arteriogram is a more uncomfortable test and consists of injecting dye not into the vein, as with most such tests, but into the artery itself. The actual point of entry in the arterial system is usually the groin. The resultant map of the arterial system is often necessary to guide subsequent surgery. Complications include the rare possibilities of an allergic dye reaction or damage to the artery.

TREATMENT

Bone Cancer

Osteogenic sarcoma is an aggressive cancer, and since it may spread through the central canal of the bone, amputation of the entire bone, as far as the next higher joint, is often required.

Chondrosarcoma, which arises from cartilage, is a slower growing and less aggressive cancer. Even though amputation is the more common procedure, in some cases surgical removal of the area involved, but not of the entire bone, may be as successful. The defect in the bone is reconstructed with bone grafts or metal prostheses.

Ewing's sarcoma, though particularly aggressive, is found in children and, before the days of modern chemotherapy, had only a 5 percent cure rate. Nowadays, after high-dose X ray or occasionally amputation of the affected bone, intensive chemotherapy is administered to destroy the cells that have already spread to the lung. Such spread virtually always occurs with this disease and has accounted for the poor cure rate without chemotherapy. With modern chemotherapy, more than half of those with Ewing's may be cured.

In fact, with Ewing's more than with osteogenic, and with osteogenic more than with chondrosarcoma, intensive chemotherapy—with the intensity of that used in leukemia—is commonplace. The chemotherapy is similar to that described below for soft tissue sarcoma.

Soft Tissue Sarcomas

The method of treatment for soft tissue sarcoma depends largely on the site of the cancer, as well as on the extent at time of diagnosis and grade. Due to the tendency of sarcomas to spread widely along anatomic structures, such as blood vessels, nerves, and muscle layers, recurrence in the same area is common. In other words, the surgeon must usually remove all the anatomic "compartment"—the whole set of muscles, bones, nerves, and/or blood vessels in the area where the tumor occurred. In the thigh, this might involve up to half the muscle. Needless to say, considerable difference in appearance, as well as a slight decrease in joint motion, and some decrease in muscular strength can be expected—at least until the remaining muscles enlarge to compensate. The change might allow for walking, but not running. Either before or after surgery, high-dose X-ray therapy might be given. The combination of two intensive treatments requires careful and complicated planning by the radiation therapist and surgeon.

In addition, depending on the likelihood of undiagnosable spread, intensive chemotherapy is often administered at the time of initial surgery. Soft tissue tumors respond markedly to chemotherapy in children, though the effect is not quite as dramatic in adults. The National Cancer Institute's program includes doxorubicin hydrochloride (Adriamycin) and cyclophosphamide (Cytoxan), begun as soon as the surgical incision has healed. When the maximal allowed dose of Adriamycin has been given—usually after eight to nine months—the chemotherapy is changed to high-dose methotrexate. Adriamycin causes permanent cardiac damage at high doses. Moreover, it causes bothersome, although not medically serious, side effects, such as temporary hairlessness. In addition, bone marrow depression, with decreases in platelets and white blood cells, as well as mouth sores and gastrointestinal cramps, may occur with virtually any chemotherapy. This is caused by chemotherapy's effect on rapidly growing tissue, such as bone marrow and the entire gastrointestinal tract, including the mouth. High-dose methotrexate must be given with much intravenous fluid, creating a large urine output, to prevent the drug's damaging the kidney and urinary tract. In addition, a medicine called citrovorum factor is also given to partially ameliorate the effect of methotrexate on normal cells. In order to monitor the high doses, blood levels of the drug are frequently checked.

Radiation has no effect on fertility unless it is aimed at the lower abdomen or pelvis, thereby causing direct damage to the ovaries. Intensive chemotherapy may damage the ovaries, especially as women approach their forties.

Other drugs—such as dacarbazine (DTIC), vincristine sulfate (Oncovin), and actinomycin D or dactinomycin—are also used in some treatment protocols.

Lymphomas (Hodgkin's Disease and Others)

L ymphoma is the general term for a large variety of cancers arising from cells in the lymphatic system. The system includes the spleen and a network of glands called lymph nodes, which are connected by small vessels that transport lymph throughout the body. Lymph is tissue fluid that circulates throughout the bloodstream. Lymphocytes, white cells that produce disease-fighting molecules called antibodies, are manufactured in the lymph nodes and spleen and enter the blood circulation through the lymph vessels.

Cancers of the lymphatic system consist of Hodgkin's disease and non-Hodgkin's lymphoma. The two often differ greatly in terms of typical patient course and expected cure rate. Hodgkin's disease is characterized by malignancies beginning in the spleen and lymph nodes. In non-Hodgkin's lymphoma, the initial site may be unknown: The area of origin in a third of the cases, or at least the site of principal involvement, is the skin, bone, and gastrointestinal tract. (Even though lymph nodes are not present in the skin, small numbers of lymph cells may reside there and may serve as a point of cancer origin.)

There are about 31,000 cases of lymphoma each year in the United States, representing 4 percent of all diagnosed cancers. Lymphomas are the seventh most common cause of cancer death in the United States. About 7,000 cases result from Hodgkin's disease, with the remaining three-quarters resulting from non-Hodgkin's lymphoma. Hodgkin's disease is rarely found in patients under the age of ten and has one period of increased incidence between ages fifteen and thirty, and another between ages seventy and eighty. Non-Hodgkin's lymphoma occurs at a later age, with about a quarter of the cases diagnosed in patients between the ages of fifty and fifty-nine, and a majority of patients diagnosed even later. Both types of lymphomas occur somewhat more commonly in males than in females, the general ratio being 1.5:1. Moreover, in the case of Hodgkin's disease, females tend to have a less aggressive cancer and respond better to treatment with a greater percentage of cure.

SYMPTOMS OF LYMPHOMA

* Enlarged lymph nodes, usually found in the neck, armpit, or groin, in that order.
* Pain and pressure in the left upper part of the abdomen, due to enlargement of the spleen.
* Night sweats.
* Weight loss.

SYMPTOMS

In Hodgkin's disease, most patients first notice painless enlarged lymph nodes. While most cases are localized to one side of the neck, the enlarged lymph node may also be in the armpit or in the groin. Occasionally, perhaps because of rapid growth, the enlarged lymph node may be slightly tender. Among patients seeking diagnosis, enlargement of neck lymph nodes will be found in 60 to 80 percent, armpit lymph nodes in 6 to 20 percent, and groin lymph nodes in 6 to 12 percent. Hodgkin's may also be diagnosed when a routine chest X ray shows enlargement of the mediastinum—the area between the two lungs, which is rich in lymph node tissue. Often mediastinal lymph node enlargement has no symptoms. On the other hand, if the enlargement is big enough to press against other structures, it may cause shortness of breath, chest tightness, or difficulty swallowing, giving the patient a sticking sensation in the midchest. On rare occasions, Hodgkin's disease starts deep in the lymph nodes of the abdomen. In that location, it may remain undiscovered for a long time, until it becomes large enough to be felt through the abdominal wall. About 30 percent of patients diagnosed with Hodgkin's have evening or night fever, often associated with much sweating and a slow weight loss. Although temperatures may be quite high, in the range of 102°F. to 104°F., patients usually do not feel ill and are able to go about their

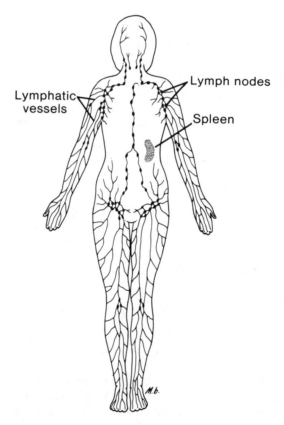

The lymphatic system

usual activities. Since there is no evidence of infection, it is felt that the fever may be caused by the tumor itself.

Non-Hodgkin's lymphomas are diagnosed with more variable symptoms than in Hodgkin's disease. The most common situation, prompting diagnosis in half the patients, involves painless enlargement of lymph nodes of both armpits, both groins, and both sides of the neck simultaneously, in contrast to involvement of only one lymph node area, which is frequently found in Hodgkin's disease. The other half of patients with non-Hodgkin's lymphoma are diagnosed with intra-abdominal enlarged lymph nodes or with the disease spread outside the nodes, usually to the skin and bone. Organ involvement at time of diagnosis may include the lung, causing shortness of breath, chest tightness, and a cough; the gastrointestinal tract, causing vomiting, gastrointestinal bleeding, and ulcerlike symptoms; the bone marrow, causing anemia, easy bruising; the central nervous system, causing headaches, paralysis, or weakness; and the skin, causing small lumps that appear to be beneath the skin. Fever, sweats, and weight loss occur in only 15 to 20 percent of patients with non-Hodgkin's lymphoma.

A large assortment of acute and chronic infectious diseases, many of them viral in nature, can cause enlargement of one lymph node, a region of lymph nodes, or all lymph nodes of the body. A common example is "swollen glands" of the neck, caused by a sore throat or abscessed teeth. Smokers often have mild long-term enlargement of the neck lymph nodes, probably from throat irritation. Marked lymph node enlargement throughout the body occurs with infectious mononucleosis. Moreover, there are people who have chronic lymph node enlargement for reasons that cannot be determined, since the lymph node biopsy shows only nonspecific increases in what appear to be normal lymphocytic cells. Long-term follow-up is important since, in as many as a third of such patients, the symptoms eventually progress, resulting in actual lymphoma.

The early stages of Hodgkin's disease, with involvement limited to one or two adjacent lymph node areas, are present in half the patients at the time of diagnosis. Patients in the early stages have a near 95 percent cure rate. Even half the patients diagnosed at a late stage appear to be cured. By contrast, more than 85 percent of patients with non-Hodgkin's lymphoma are diagnosed at late stages, with generalized lymph node involvement or involvement of nonlymphatic organs, such as the liver, lung, or bones. The average five-year survival of all patients with non-Hodgkin's lymphoma is about 30 percent, which probably reflects its more aggressive nature and diagnosis at a later stage.

WHO IS AT RISK?

Both exposure to radiation and previous diseases of the immune system cause an increased rate of lymphoma. The survivors of the atomic bomb in Hiroshima show an increased incidence of most kinds of lymphoma. Long-term follow-up of British men who received large doses of irradiation for a nonmalignant spinal disease also showed increased incidence of lymphoma. In both studies, the number of actual cases was twice that which occurred in similar persons not exposed to radiation. The so-called autoimmune diseases—such as lupus, Sjögren's syndrome, and rheumatoid arthritis—predispose a patient to development of lymphoma. Patients with long-standing Sjögren's syndrome—a condition causing dry eyes, dry mouth, and joint disease, occurring in 1 to 2 percent of women—have almost a 10 percent chance of developing lymphoma during their lifetime.

There is no familial predisposition to lymphoma. For a time, an infectious agent, causing spread by contagion, was suspected in Hodgkin's disease. Suspicion arose after one particular report involving the clustering of several cases in some school buildings. However, there has been no further confirmation of such a theory. Moreover, medical personnel who specialize in the treatment of patients with lymphoma do not have a higher incidence of the disease.

Despite overwhelming evidence of the viral cause of animal lymphoma and the contagious nature of lymphosarcomas in cats, chickens, and cows, there is no proof of a viral, or any other contagious, agent in human lymphoma. On the other hand, the inability to establish a viral cause in human lymphoma—as has been done in animal lymphoma—may be due to the limitations of research. Developing inbred strains and obtaining fetal tissue, while important in animal research, is impossible with human subjects.

DIAGNOSIS

Diagnosis of lymphoma generally involves removal of an enlarged lymph node, a minor surgical procedure that can usually be performed in the physician's office or in an outpatient clinic setting. Occasionally, the procedure may require general anesthesia and a short hospitalization. Removal of the entire node, rather than part, is necessary, since lymphoma classifications often require study of the entire lymph node architecture as well as of the abnormal cells themselves. Sometimes the first node removed is abnormal, but not abnormal enough to make a diagnosis certain. In those cases, a second lymph node biopsy is required several weeks or a month later. If the mediastinum is the site of enlarged lymph nodes, sufficient tissue can sometimes be removed through a one-inch neck incision, a procedure called mediastinoscopy. (See the description of that procedure in the section on lung cancer.)

Although lymph node biopsies are the most common method of diagnosis for both Hodgkin's disease and non-Hodgkin's lymphoma, skin or bone nodules are sometimes biopsied in non-Hodgkin's lymphoma. The treatment of Hodgkin's disease and non-Hodgkin's lymphoma depends not only on the extent of the disease but in some cases also on the specific subtype. Accordingly, even if the microscopic picture is classical for a particular subtype, it is safest to have the slides examined by an experienced hematopathologist for confirmation.

As mentioned, there are many reasons for individual or generalized lymph node enlargement, particularly in the adolescent and early adult years. Most reasons involve viral infections, such as the flu and mononucleosis. Therefore, it is important that any lymph node—

whether in the neck, armpit, or groin—remaining enlarged after the other symptoms of the infection have disappeared be evaluated by a physician for possible biopsy.

STAGING AND TREATMENT

Hodgkin's Disease

Hodgkin's disease is treated by both X rays and drugs. Since therapy is specifically tailored to the extent of the disease, numerous tests are routinely employed to confirm the stage. For example, if a patient were diagnosed with neck lymph node involvement alone, the treatment would be X-ray therapy to that area and the area immediately adjacent, because Hodgkin's disease is thought to spread in an orderly manner from one lymph node group to the next adjacent one.

A careful chest X ray and CT scan of the chest are sometimes necessary to determine mediastinal lymph node enlargement. If lymph nodes in other areas of the body are enlarged, they may also be biopsied to determine their true nature. Bone marrow aspiration under local anesthesia (a procedure described fully in the section on leukemia) will usually be performed. Samples will be taken from both the right and left pelvic bones. This is more important in non-Hodgkin's lymphoma, where 10 to 20 percent of cases involve the bone marrow, than in Hodgkin's disease, with its 1 percent involvement.

Many of the body's lymph nodes are located in the back of the abdomen with the great vessels. The lymphangiogram has been the standard means of evaluating spread in this area. In a lymphangiogram, X-ray dye is injected into a lymphatic vessel of each foot. Within twenty-four hours, the dye has traveled up the leg and outlined the groin, or inguinal, lymph nodes, the pelvic lymph nodes, and some of the lymph nodes lying along the aorta (the largest artery). The dye uniformly stains the normal lymph nodes, while the abnormal areas remain unstained. The CT scan of the abdomen supplements the lymphangiogram, and sometimes may even replace it.

Sometimes a laparoscopy—an evaluation by a scope through a one-inch incision—is performed, along with a liver biopsy, to determine the spread of the disease. Unfortunately, the spleen, which is part of the lymphatic system and may be diseased, and important lymph node areas in the back of the abdomen cannot be visualized with this technique, so the place of laparoscopy in the staging of lymphoma is limited. (See the section on ovarian cancer for a description of this procedure.)

If an exploratory laparotomy will significantly aid the physician in determining the kind of chemotherapy or radiation treatment the patient should receive, it is performed to visualize and examine the lymph nodes and organs. Several lymph node areas and both lobes of the liver are biopsied, and the spleen is removed—all for microscopic analysis and staging. The diagnosis of Stage I lymphoma is limited to involvement of a single group of lymph nodes in one area of the body, such as the neck or the armpit. Stage II involves two lymph node areas, adjacent to each other and both in the upper or lower half of the body, the dividing line being the diaphragm. Stage III involves both the lymph node regions on either side of the diaphragm (such as neck and groin) and the spleen. Stage IV entails diffuse spread outside the lymphatic system and often includes the liver and bone marrow. As mentioned, many staging tests are necessary to determine the precise extent, and subsequent treatment, of the disease. Too little treatment could result in failure to cure the disease, while extensive treatment results in unnecessary side effects.

In general, a Stage I or II patient receives X-ray therapy in the area called the mantle. If the patient is Stage I or II, but also has had fever, night sweats, and weight loss, more extensive treatment, sometimes involving chemotherapy, is required. For a greater extent of disease, total nodal radiotherapy may be administered. "Total nodal" is actually a misnomer in that it does not treat all the lymph nodes of the body. It consists of X-ray treatment to the mantle area, the inverted Y, and the spleen. A patient might have the mantle area irradiated over six weeks, rest a month, and then return for X-ray therapy to the inverted Y over the next six weeks. The complications of such X-ray treatment may include radiation damage to the lung and lining of the heart, as well as prolonged decreases in red cell, white cell, and platelet counts caused by extensive irradiation of the bone marrow. Temporary or permanent ovarian failure with sterility usually accompanies inverted Y radiation.

Chemotherapy for Hodgkin's disease is often a regimen called MOPP: nitrogen mustard (Mustargen), vincristine sulfate (Oncovin), procarbazine hydrochloride (Matulane), and prednisone. First used in 1967, it resulted in a 55 percent, five-year survival rate for late-stage Hodgkin's disease. While this combination remains the standard, several others have shown similar results. Several months of chemotherapy is often the usual course.

Chemotherapy produces the usual side effects of nausea and vomiting, though there is little hair loss. Men are often rendered sterile by intensive chemotherapy of any kind. Before starting such a program, sperm can be frozen and stored for later use. Young women may experience ovarian dysfunction during chemotherapy, with intermittent spotting instead of regular periods. However, ovarian function usually returns to normal when the drug is stopped, and fertility is often

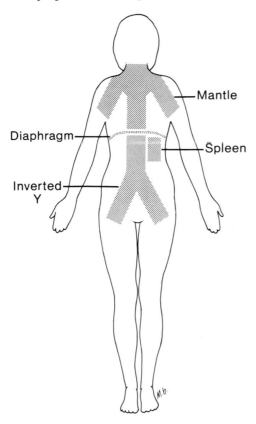

Labels: Mantle, Diaphragm, Spleen, Inverted Y

Radiation treatment areas in lymphoma

retained. The younger the woman, the fewer the problems with subsequent fertility. Women in their thirties are at greater risk for infertility, since the older ovary is more vulnerable to permanent chemotherapeutic damage. Nevertheless, if a woman can become pregnant, there should be little or no problem with continuing the pregnancy and delivering. If a woman is in her forties, chemotherapy may produce premature menopause.

Regrettably, cancer treatment can also cause cancer. In patients receiving both X ray and drugs for Hodgkin's disease, 5 percent develop non-Hodgkin's lymphoma within ten years. However, it is clear that prior to the development of X-ray treatments and chemotherapy 95 percent of the Hodgkin's patients requiring such treatment died within five years.

Non-Hodgkin's Lymphoma

Since most non-Hodgkin's lymphomas are in advanced stages when diagnosed, combination chemotherapy is almost always used. At the same time, the less serious types may do well for years with single-drug chemotherapy and even, though rarely, with no treatment at all. Localized X-ray therapy is often used for shrinking tumors and palliating symptoms, even if cure is not possible. Prior to chemotherapy, surgery may be necessary to treat gastrointestinal lymphomas for complications caused by tumor growth, such as bowel obstruction, perforation, and bleeding.

Treatment and expected survival depend significantly on microscopic subtype: nodular, which refers to the preservation of the lymph node's normal structure, and diffuse, which indicates that the normal structure has become unrecognizable due to extensive infiltration of malignant cells. There is a large division between the nodular types, which are less aggressive, and the diffuse, which are more so.

For the nodular subtypes of non-Hodgkin's lymphoma, the chemotherapy might involve a regimen called COP: cyclophosphamide (Cytoxan), vincristine sulfate (Oncovin), and prednisone. Chlorambucil (Leukeran) and prednisone are sometimes used, especially in older patients. After a long slow-moving or even stationary phase of several years or a decade in duration, the nodular non-Hodgkin's lymphoma may progress quickly, often becoming resistant to chemotherapy. When this occurs, the microscopic appearance often changes to that of a diffuse lymphoma.

Before the development of aggressive chemotherapy, patients diagnosed with diffuse lymphomas had an average survival of two years. However, with chemotherapy, often consisting of cyclophosphamide, vincristine sulfate, and prednisone with procarbazine, Adriamycin, or bleomycin sulfate, there is a complete remission rate of 60 to 80 percent. Of those achieving complete remission, the majority survive for several years and many appear cured.

The side effects from chemotherapy for non-Hodgkin's disease range from mild, with chlorambucil and prednisone, to more troublesome with stronger agents. Besides nausea, vomiting, mouth sores, and hair loss, side effects may include the production of a large amount of uric acid, which can cause uric acid stones in the kidneys. These are treated by increased fluid intake and by drugs that change the acidity of the urine, which helps uric acid dissolve. Low red cell, white cell, and platelet counts may also result from the bone marrow damage of chemotherapy.

Leukemia

L eukemia (literally, "white blood") is a form of cancer in which malignant white blood cells rapidly reproduce themselves. White blood cells, or leukocytes, are actually not white but colorless. They are found in the bloodstream and, to an even greater extent, elsewhere in the body: in the lymph nodes, connective tissue, and tissue spaces of various organs. White blood cells possess a certain degree of mobility and, like amoebas, can squeeze through spaces too small for a red blood cell and thus leave the bloodstream. For every white cell in the circulating blood, there are more than 500 red blood cells—or, to put it another way, there are normally 5,000 to 9,000 white blood cells per cubic millimeter of normal circulating blood. In leukemia, leukocytes sometimes reach a level of several hundred thousand per cubic millimeter.

The white cells are divided into three groups: granulocytes, which destroy bacteria that would cause infections; lymphocytes, which are responsible for the immune response; and monocytes, which destroy foreign material, but not necessarily bacteria, that may enter the body. Granulocytes, named for the granules they contain, are formed in the bone marrow, along with red blood cells and platelets, and account for three-quarters of white blood cells. Most of them act as scavengers, engulfing and removing foreign material from the blood and tissue spaces. Other granulocytes take part in the allergic reaction. When there is an invasion of bacteria into the tissues, as through a skin cut, great numbers of granulocytes flow through the bloodstream toward the site and then pass through the blood vessel walls into the fluid between the cells. The bacteria are walled off by granulocytes, a process resulting in pus formation. As their name suggests, lymphocytes are associated with lymph, a fluid that eventually enters the bloodstream, carrying lymphocytes with it. Lymphocytes constitute 20 percent of white blood cells in the bloodstream and produce the protein antibodies important in immunologic functioning. Monocytes, which have an undefined role in immunologic function, comprise only 2 percent. Unlike granulocytes, neither lymphocytes nor monocytes have the ability to engulf and destroy bacteria and other foreign cells.

Bone marrow, the liquid fatty material located in the hollow center of most large bones, is responsible for manufacturing most blood cells, including the red cells (for carrying oxygen), platelets (for clotting blood), and certain white cells. Some white blood cells, particularly the lymphocytes, are formed not in the bone marrow but in the lymphoid tissue of the lymph nodes, spleen, liver, and in several other organs. However, since many of them eventually find their way into the bloodstream, they are considered together with other white blood cells. Leukemias are divided into the acute and chronic forms. Leukemia originating from granulocyte cells can be called granulocytic, but more often it is named after the location in which it is formed: myeloid, myelocytic, myelogenous are all names referring to the bone marrow, the common site of granulocyte development. Leukemia originating from lymphocytes is called lymphocytic or lymphoblastic. (Monocytes are rarely, if ever, the cell of origin of leukemia.) Actually, most acute leukemias (whether myelogenous or lymphocytic in origin) resemble one another, as do chronic leukemias.

For most cancers, striking differences in frequency exist from country to country. This is considerably less the case for leukemia than for other forms of cancer, with little more than a twofold difference between the United States and any country with comparably reliable reporting.

As with other cancers, the rate of leukemia occurrence varies with age. Overall annual incidence rises with age from a low of 1 to 2 cases per 100,000 in young adulthood to 30 or more cases per 100,000 in people over fifty. Approximately 8,000 new cases of acute adult leukemia were diagnosed in the United States in 1984. An additional 13,000 to 14,000 patients developed chronic leukemia, with approximately equal division between granulocytic and lymphocytic types. Leukemia is not among the five most common causes of cancer deaths, but in the subgroup of patients between fifteen and thirty-four years, it is the leading cause in men and is second only to breast cancer in women. Males are generally more often affected by leukemia than are females, with a ratio of two men to every woman. Overall, leukemia affects many more adults than children, with half of all leukemias occurring in persons over sixty. Unlike most other cancers, however, a distinct childhood peak exists, rising to about 5 cases per 100,000 at two to four years of age and decreasing in later childhood.

Acute Leukemias—Lymphocytic and Myelogenous

Acute leukemias are intense diseases and may run their course in several weeks or months. The predominant leukemia of childhood is acute lymphocytic leukemia where the involved cell originates from the lymphocyte. This disease is rarely found in people over the age of fifteen; most of the leukemia diagnosed is acute myelogenous leukemia (AML), occurring mainly between the ages of fifteen and fifty-five. Complete remission—meaning that all symptoms disappear—can be effected in adults 60 to 70 percent of the time. However, the overall outlook for cure in adults with acute leukemia is not as good as in children.

Chronic Leukemia

Chronic leukemias may run their course in years, or even decades. Chronic granulocytic leukemia, usually called chronic myelogenous leukemia ("myelo" means bone marrow), originates in the granulocyte, one of the most important cells for fighting infection. This disease occurs most often in persons between the ages of forty and sixty.

Chronic lymphocytic leukemia (CLL) is a disease of older persons—those in their fifties, sixties, and seventies. This disease can be slowly progressive, making its presence known with enlargement of the lymph nodes or spleen, though often with no other symptoms. The course of this disease is more variable than with other leukemias.

SYMPTOMS OF LEUKEMIA

- Fatigue and weakness.
- Fever and chills.
- Weight loss.
- Easy bruising.
- Bone and joint pain.
- Pain and pressure in the left upper part of the abdomen, due to enlargement of the spleen.

SYMPTOMS

The signs of acute leukemia are directly related to the elimination of normal blood cells by leukemic cells. Interference with production of red cells causes anemia, which, in turn, causes paleness of the skin, fatigue, and shortness of breath. Quickened pulse and heart strain can also occur as the blood must be more rapidly pumped to compensate for the lack of oxygen. Lack of platelet production causes bleeding of the gums, nose bleeds, easy bruising, blood in the urine, rectal bleeding, or bleeding into any internal organ. The leukemic white blood cells, while they may be numerous, are so abnormal that they do not perform normal functions, such as engulfing bacteria or producing antibodies. Lack of production of the normal white cells that fight infection can cause sore throats, mouth sores, pneumonia, and urinary infections, usually associated with an elevated temperature. Pressure from the leukemic cell deposits may cause aching pains over the bones, particularly those of the arms, legs, or the spine, where the large bone marrow cavities are located. The mass of white cells can even clog the blood vessels. Upon diagnosis, 90 percent of patients experience fatigue and weakness; 80 percent, fever and/or chills with or without an obvious infection; 50 percent, weight loss; 30 to 50 percent, evidence of easy bruising; and 25 percent, bone and joint pain.

The signs of chronic leukemia are more slowly progressive and hence more subtle. Many patients have no symptoms, but are found to have too many white blood cells—granulocytes in the case of chronic granulocytic (myelogenous) leukemia or lymphocytes in the case of chronic lymphocytic leukemia—on a routine blood count done for other purposes, such as hospital admission for hernia repair or hysterectomy. Some patients notice lack of energy and are easily fatigued. The only common specific finding is a hard swelling of the left part of the upper abdomen, usually painless, caused by the marked enlargement of the spleen. On occasion, the spleen enlargement may be massive, extending down to the navel, and associated with pain and pressure from its weight and surface inflammation.

WHO IS AT RISK?

Despite their rarity, comprising only 5 percent of cancers in the United States, leukemias have been studied more extensively than many other cancers. This is partly due to the fact that they involve tissue systems—blood and marrow—that are easily accessible for diagnosis, monitoring, and research studies. In fact, not only are leukemic cells especially accessible for sampling, but the leukemic cells can be separated more readily from normal cells to make a purer cancer cell mixture than is possible with solid tumors, such as breast or colon. The ability to examine and study pure preparations of malignant cells is a great advantage in research.

In contrast to other human cancers, research in leukemia has also been greatly facilitated by animal models in which leukemias occur (mice, rats, birds, cows, cats, and monkeys). Nonetheless, research in leukemia has not yet progressed to where guidelines exist for its prevention. Only in the cases of ionizing radiation and the chemical benzene is exposure known to cause leukemia.

X Rays

X rays have long been known to cause leukemia. The earliest evidence consisted of cases arising in radiation workers soon after the discovery of X rays early in this century. Subsequently, it was shown that radiologists were nine times more likely to have leukemia than the nonradiologist physicians in the 1930s and 1940s. This excess has decreased in recent decades, presumably as safeguards improved.

Considerable research has focused on three kinds of human exposure: nuclear reactions, medical radiation therapy, and X rays for medical diagnosis. Whatever the source, two factors need to be emphasized. First, an increased incidence of leukemia is related to increased radiation dose. Second, periods from two or three years to twenty or more years can be expected between exposure to radiation and the onset of the disease.

Study of the Japanese population exposed to atomic bomb radiation showed increases in all kinds of leukemia (except chronic lymphocytic), with the earliest cases appearing about two years after the bomb and the peak between five and ten years. The younger the person exposed to the radiation, the shorter the period between radiation exposure and the appearance of leukemia. And, of course, the higher the dose, the greater the risk.

Strong evidence exists for radiation-induced leukemia in persons who received therapeutic X-ray treatments for various diseases. Evidence of increased leukemia following X rays for diagnostic, rather than for treatment, purposes appears in studies of offspring of mothers who received X rays during pregnancy. The increased sensitivity of rapidly dividing fetal cells is believed to account for the X ray's ability to cause leukemia, even at very small doses. Surprisingly, X-ray exposure after the fetal stage has not been proven to cause leukemia—probably because the common X-ray doses are small, adults are less susceptible, and, given the rarity of the disease, a few extra cases are difficult to detect.

Chemical and Drug Exposure

Of the various chemicals, only benzene (an organic solvent) is known as an agent that probably increases the risk of leukemia. Occupations that involve benzene are leather and shoe manufacturing, dry cleaning, printing, and painting. The leukemia is often preceded by abnormally low blood counts for several years, indicating damage to the bone marrow, which may either reverse itself or progress to leukemia.

Certain chemotherapeutic drugs have also been implicated in causing leukemia, with an estimated fifty-fold increase in the expected occurrence for persons who have required these drugs. This means that the risk for each individual will rise to about 1 per 1,000 and is, therefore, still quite small. The drugs accounting for 75 percent of chemotherapy-induced leukemias are melphalan (Alkeran), chlorambucil (Leukeran), azathioprine (Imuran), and Thiotepa. Less suspect drugs are vinblastine sulfate (Velban), nitrogen mustard (Mustargen), methotrexate, and fluorouracil (5-FU). Of course, patients treated with both X-ray therapy and these drugs have an even higher risk than those treated with one alone.

Viruses—a Cause?

Infectious agents, such as viruses, may also play a role in human leukemia. The viral cause of animal leukemia has been repeatedly demonstrated. Lacking the possibility of the same kinds of experimental studies on man as are conducted with animals, researchers must use indirect means to investigate viruses in human leukemias. Considerable work has been devoted to the theory that animal leukemia viruses are infectious and may at least partly account for the occurrence of human leukemia. However, blood studies of animal keepers who happen to develop leukemia showed no evidence of the animal virus. Animal owners and animal workers do not have higher rates of leukemia.

Over the past twenty years, researchers have studied whether leukemia occurs "in clusters" from persons in contact with each other, thereby reflecting the passage of viral or other infectious agents that are as yet unidentified. The conclusion has been that there is no tendency for cases to cluster. Specifically, there is no tendency for leukemia to occur with greater frequency in spouses of leukemia patients, in children born to leukemic mothers, or in persons who receive blood transfusions from individuals who develop leukemia.

There is no genetic or familial predisposition in adult leukemias. Persons with some chromosomal diseases, such as Down's and Fanconi syndromes, are prone to leukemias.

Preventive Measures

As concerns chemicals, prevention must focus on minimizing contact with benzene in the various industries named. People outside these occupations might come into contact with benzene only as a gasoline additive. One should certainly avoid breathing gasoline fumes.

One should avoid unnecessary irradiation, and certainly no pregnant woman should be X-rayed unless absolutely necessary because of the leukemia risk to the offspring.

DIAGNOSIS

The first step in diagnosis is a complete blood count that allows for the visualization and identification of the malignant white cells. In most patients with acute leukemia, the number of red cells transporting oxygen is severely decreased, and the number of platelets, responsible for clotting, is also below normal. In the chronic leukemias, the decrease in red cells and platelets is usually minimal, if it occurs at all.

Bone Marrow Aspiration

The next step, bone marrow aspiration (removal of a specimen of bone marrow using a syringe and needle), is performed in the patient's hospital room or in the doctor's office. The sample usually comes from the side (ileum) or back (sacrum) of the pelvic bone. The patient is positioned on her stomach or side, depending on the specific bone to be aspirated. The area overlying the bone is cleansed with antiseptic liquid and draped in a sterile manner. The skin, fat, and lining over the bone are locally anesthetized. The patient usually feels pain during injection of the local anesthetic and pain to a smaller extent when the needle is inserted into the bone, a procedure that requires considerable pressure. A sharp, quick pain may be felt during the actual aspiration in which the syringe plunger is drawn back to extract a teaspoon's worth of the bone marrow specimen. Microscopic examination reveals the number, size, and shape of the red blood cells, white blood cells, and platelets, as these cells evolve through various stages of development in the bone marrow. The rare complications of bone marrow biopsy or aspiration are relatively minor and include excessive bleeding, infection, and puncture of a blood vessel. For a bone and bone marrow biopsy, a biopsy instrument is screwed into the bone through a small incision, allowing removal of a tiny fragment of the bone itself for analysis.

TREATMENT

Acute Leukemia

CHEMOTHERAPY. The treatment for leukemia is chemotherapy. It aims at destroying all the leukemic white blood cells, which may number as many as one trillion (10^{18}) at the time of diagnosis. Four out of five adult patients achieve complete remission, which is specifically defined as disappearance of all symptoms, with no leukemic cells detectable in the blood or bone marrow, and no lingering side effects from chemotherapy. Unfortunately, this does not always mean cure. There may still be as many as 100 million leukemic cells present even if the blood and bone marrow appear to be normal. This is the number that would still remain, for example, even if the treatment killed 99.99 percent of the leukemic cells.

There is a likelihood that cells can become resistant to the drugs over a period of given use. Accordingly, induction chemotherapy involves the administration of multiple drugs in high doses, but only for short durations. The treatment requires hospitalization in a specialized facility to treat the expected side effects. Maintenance therapy for two years or so is given to a patient in complete remission to prevent regrowth of leukemic cells. Maintenance treatment is less intense, with far fewer side effects, and is given on an outpatient basis.

For the 10 to 15 percent of adults with the lymphocytic variety of acute leukemias, a chemotherapy program might include use of vincristine sulfate (Oncovin), asparaginase (Elspar), and prednisone. About 70 to 80 percent will achieve complete remission. Even as remission continues, the brain and spinal cord may be the site of recurrence in half of all patients, since most chemotherapy drugs are blood-borne drugs and do not penetrate the cerebrospinal fluid. Accordingly, the brain and spine are often irradiated at some point, or chemotherapy is injected directly into the spinal fluid.

In the 85 to 90 percent of adults with the myeloid variety of acute leukemia, the treatment is also chemotherapy. Before chemotherapy was developed, patients averaged two to four months of survival. Now, a quarter of adults who achieve complete remission are cured. Usually, drugs such as daunorubicin hydrochloride (Cerubidine), cytosine arabinoside (Cytosar-V), and sometimes 6-thioguanine are given in high doses over the first seven days of hospitalization.

There are profound side effects, which include hair loss, severe nausea, and vomiting. More serious still are the metabolic abnormalities—high blood levels of uric acid, calcium, and phosphate—caused by the breakdown products of the cells. These abnormalities necessitate careful monitoring and treatment. About seven to ten days after treatment, the white cell, red cell, and platelet counts have dropped to their lowest point, and intensive skilled support is necessary, since patients are susceptible to life-threatening infections and bleeding. Following this, there is rapid and complete recovery of bone marrow function and the cell counts return to normal levels. After induction therapy, most patients spend twenty to forty days in the hospital before returning home. If complete remission has been achieved, the patient may continue with maintenance therapy.

BONE MARROW TRANSPLANT. Another promising new procedure is bone marrow transplant, in which healthy bone marrow from a close relative with a similar genetic makeup is injected into the bone marrow spaces of the leukemic patient. The actual transfer of the bone marrow is performed under sterile conditions in the operating room, with the donor under general anesthesia. Before the transplant, chemotherapy and X-ray doses strong enough to destroy all the bone marrow—cancerous and normal—are given to the leukemic patient. The treatment destroys the production of red blood cells, white blood cells, and platelets, until the donated bone marrow can establish itself and produce adequate normal cells. During these several weeks, the patient is kept in a sterile hospital environment and even eats sterilized food until the new bone marrow is well established and functioning properly. Failure of the donated bone marrow to grow, while rare, is often a fatal complication. Another complication involves attack of the patient's own cells by the cells produced in the donated bone marrow. This can produce problems in the skin, gastrointestinal tract, and liver.

Bone marrow transplant is so intense and difficult to withstand that only leukemic patients who are otherwise in excellent medical condition are considered for treatment. For whatever reason, it is mainly patients with acute myelogenous leukemia, rather than with acute lymphocytic leukemia, who have done well with bone marrow transplants. Also, the leukemic patient must have a compatible brother or sister willing to donate his or her bone marrow. Statistically, there is only a 25 percent chance that a sibling will have compatible tissue. As far as the donor is concerned, the procedure may be thought similar to giving blood for a transfusion. There is abundant bone marrow remaining, and the donor suffers no immediate or long-term side effects from donation. In fact, the donated marrow sites are merely multiple needle punctures that heal without scars. About half the transplant patients survive long-term and may be cured, to judge from the as yet brief follow-up of most patients.

Chronic Myelocytic (Granulocytic) Leukemia

The initial treatment for patients with chronic myelocytic leukemia is mild, usually consisting of busulfan (Myleran) or hydroxyurea (Hydrea) administered by pill taken daily as an outpatient. The leukemic cell count is monitored with weekly blood tests until it drops to normal, which often requires three to four weeks of the daily dosage. Somewhat more slowly than the white cell count decreases, the spleen gradually shrinks, and maximum improvement here may take three months. Maintenance therapy is then started with the same drug at a decreased dose, usually given once or twice a week. Unfortunately, the "chronic" phase eventually ends and the "blast" phase begins. Immature cells, or blasts, are then made and released in great numbers, with results similar to those of acute leukemia. This stage is less treatable than acute leukemia.

Although incurable, the disease is controllable for many years, sometimes as long as ten, with the average survival about five years. Until progression occurs, patients usually have no symptoms and are able to work and enjoy a normal life. Patients with chronic granulocytic leukemia are older, and many die of other diseases while their leukemia is in check. The chemotherapy involved in induction and maintenance is milder than many others, though it may cause darkening of the skin.

Chronic Lymphocytic Leukemia

Chronic lymphocytic leukemia is closely related to the lymphomas—most patients have enlarged lymph nodes—and in some cases may have progressed from what was previously diagnosed as lymphoma. Sometimes, the only difference between this disease and lymphoma is the involvement of the bone marrow in the case of chronic lymphocytic leukemia. Nevertheless, the diagnosis is based on the appearance of abnormal white blood cells (lymphocytes in this instance) in the blood and sometimes in the marrow. For this reason it is considered a blood cancer, a leukemia.

Many patients have a slow course of the disease, including no progression of symptoms for many years. It is best not to treat such patients until true symptoms develop, since early treatment will not prevent the disease from worsening. When a patient develops a low red cell or platelet count, weight loss, fever, or enlarged lymph nodes or spleen, treatment will usually commence. The initial treatment is mild, consisting, in some cases, of only prednisone (a steroid agent) by pill; alternatively, it may be combined with chlorambucil by pill for several days twice a month. The maintenance treatment may be continued for a year; then all drugs may be stopped until symptoms reappear, perhaps several months or years later. If and when the symptoms return, the same induction may be given.

If a patient has only a high lymphocyte count in the blood, average survival is ten years, though some patients live twenty years or more. If a patient is diagnosed with a high lymphocyte count, as well as with enlarged lymph nodes, spleen, and liver, the average survival is somewhat less. But since most patients are older, they may die of other causes first.

After a Cure

Because such intensive therapy (particularly bone marrow transplant) is so recent, the aftereffects of chemotherapy for leukemia on the fertility and childbearing ability of women have not been completely determined. In general, the older the woman who undergoes chemotherapy, the more likely she is to be rendered infertile, therefore, only a small percentage of those in their teens will be rendered infertile. Women in their thirties and forties will experience a greater effect on ovarian function, including possible premature menopause. However, if a woman is able to become pregnant, even if she is in her late thirties, the previous chemotherapy should not interfere with the ability to continue the pregnancy and deliver. In other words, chemotherapy affects ovarian function most of all, but should not significantly interfere with other reproductive organ functioning. And, as mentioned, children of leukemic mothers are not at increased risk of developing leukemia.

Bibliography

Levitt, P. M., and E. S. Guralnick. *The Cancer Reference Book: Direct and Clear Answers to Everyone's Questions.* Paddington Press, 1979.

Lynch, Henry T., M.D., ed. *Cancer and You.* Springfield, IL: C. C. Thomas, 1971.

McKhann, Charles F., M.D. *The Facts About Cancer: A Guide for Patients, Family and Friends.* Englewood Cliffs, NJ: Prentice-Hall, 1981.

Mora, Marion, and Eve Potts. *Choices: Realistic Alternatives in Cancer Treatment.* New York: Avon Books, 1980.

Murphy, Gerald P., M.D., ed. *Cancer: Signals and Safeguards.* Littleton, MA: PSG Publishing Co., 1981.

Pagana, Kathleen D., and Timothy J. Pagana, M.D. *Understanding Medical Testing.* St. Louis: Plume Books of the Mosby Medical Library, 1983.

Rosenbaum, Ernest H., M.D. *Living With Cancer.* St. Louis: Plume Books of the Mosby Medical Library, 1983.

Salsbury, Kathryn H., and Eleanor L. Johnson. *The Indispensable Cancer Handbook.* NY: Seaview Books, 1981.

Watson, Rita E., and Robert C. Wallach, M.D. *New Choices, New Changes: A Woman's Guide to Conquering Cancer.* New York: St. Martin's Press, 1981.

Index